The Heart-Healthy Cookbook

100 Delicious and Nutritious Recipes for a Healthy Heart

COPYRIGHT

All rights reserved.

No part of this book may be reproduced in any form or by any electronic or mechanical means, including information storage and retrieval systems, without permission in writing from the publisher, except by a reviewer who may quote brief passages in a review.

The information contained in this book is based on the author's research and experience. While the author has made every effort to provide accurate and up-to-date information, errors and omissions may occur. The author and publisher assume no responsibility for any errors or omissions or for any actions taken based on the information contained in this book.

The information contained in this book is provided "as is," without warranty of any kind, express or implied, including but not limited to the warranties of merchantability, fitness for a particular purpose, or non-infringement. In no event shall the author or publisher be liable for any claim, damages, or other liability, whether in an action of contract, tort, or otherwise, arising from, out of, or in connection with the book or the use or other dealings in the book.

TABLE OF CONTENTS

INTRODUCTION

In the rhythmic cadence of life, our hearts beat a steadfast rhythm, orchestrating the symphony of our existence. This vital organ is the linchpin of our well-being, tirelessly pumping life through our veins. It's a masterpiece of nature, and it deserves our utmost care. With every beat, it propels life-giving blood throughout our veins, ensuring the nourishment of our cells and the vitality of our being. But, like a delicate instrument, the heart is susceptible to the rhythms of life we play, and its health hinges upon the notes we strike in our daily choices.

The importance of heart-healthy cooking cannot be overstated. Your culinary decisions have a direct and profound impact on the well-being of this vital organ, and by extension, on your overall quality of life. Each ingredient you choose, every recipe you prepare, and every meal you savor shapes the destiny of your cardiovascular health.

In this comprehensive guide, we embark on a journey to discover the path to a healthier heart through the art of cooking. Whether you're an individual striving to prevent heart disease, someone living with a heart condition, or simply a health-conscious food lover, this guide is designed to be your compass, your source of inspiration, and your trusted companion on the road to a robust, resilient heart.

We begin by delving into the intricacies of heart disease, demystifying its various forms, and unveiling the risk factors that make it a formidable adversary. Knowledge is the first step towards empowerment. We break down the essential components of a heart-healthy diet, providing you with a clear blueprint for making the right food choices. Learn about the nutrients that fuel your heart's well-being.

Discover the art of meal planning, a crucial tool for maintaining a heart-healthy diet. We guide you through portion control and the balance that ensures you eat with purpose and moderation. Explore the vast array of heart-healthy ingredients that can transform your culinary creations. Your kitchen is your laboratory for nourishment. We'll equip you with the knowledge to make the most of it, introducing heart-friendly cooking techniques and practical tips.

With this guide as your companion, you'll not only develop a profound understanding of heart-healthy cooking but also acquire practical skills and recipes that will allow you to savor delicious, nourishing meals. You'll come to appreciate the joy that cooking for your heart can bring, for the path to a healthier heart is not one of deprivation, but rather one of empowerment, delight, and boundless culinary exploration.

CHAPTER ONE

Understanding heart disease and its risk factors is fundamental to making informed choices about heart-healthy cooking and lifestyle. Heart disease, also known as cardiovascular disease, encompasses a range of conditions that affect the heart and blood vessels. It is a leading cause of morbidity and mortality worldwide, but with the right knowledge and preventive measures, it can often be managed or even prevented. Let's explore the basics of heart disease and the common risk factors associated with it:

I. Types of Heart Disease:

• Coronary Artery Disease (CAD): CAD is the most common form of heart disease. It occurs when the coronary arteries, responsible for supplying blood to the heart muscle, become narrowed or blocked by a buildup of plaque (atherosclerosis). This can lead to chest pain (angina) and heart attacks.

• Heart Failure: Heart failure occurs when the heart can't pump blood effectively, leading to symptoms like fatigue, shortness of breath, and swelling. It can result from various heart conditions.

• Arrhythmias: These are abnormal heart rhythms, which can be too fast (tachycardia) or too slow (bradycardia). They can lead to palpitations, dizziness, and fainting.

• Valvular Heart Disease: This involves problems with the heart's valves, such as stenosis (narrowing) or regurgitation (leakage), which can disrupt blood flow.

• Cardiomyopathy: Cardiomyopathy is a disease of the heart muscle that affects its ability to pump effectively.

• Congenital Heart Defects: Some individuals are born with structural heart abnormalities that may require surgical intervention.

II. Common Risk Factors for Heart Disease:

• High Blood Pressure (Hypertension): Elevated blood pressure puts additional strain on the heart and blood vessels, increasing the risk of heart disease.

• High Cholesterol: High levels of LDL ("bad") cholesterol and low levels of HDL ("good") cholesterol can contribute to the buildup of plaque in the arteries.

• Smoking: Smoking damages blood vessels, decreases oxygen in the blood, and increases the risk of atherosclerosis and blood clot formation.

• Diabetes: People with diabetes are at greater risk of heart disease due to elevated blood sugar levels that can damage blood vessels.

• Obesity: Excess body weight, especially around the abdomen, can lead to metabolic syndrome, increasing the risk of heart disease.

• Physical Inactivity: A sedentary lifestyle can contribute to weight gain and worsen other heart disease risk factors.

• Unhealthy Diet: A diet high in saturated and trans fats, cholesterol, sodium, and added sugars can lead to obesity, high blood pressure, and high cholesterol.

• Family History: A family history of heart disease can increase your risk.

• Age: The risk of heart disease increases with age.

• Gender: Men are generally at higher risk for heart disease than premenopausal women. However, the risk becomes more equal after menopause.

• Stress: Chronic stress can contribute to heart disease through various mechanisms, including unhealthy coping behaviors.

• Alcohol Consumption: Excessive alcohol consumption can lead to high blood pressure, heart failure, and other heart-related issues.

Understanding these risk factors is the first step in preventing heart disease. By making informed dietary choices, adopting a heart-healthy lifestyle, and seeking regular medical check-ups, individuals can significantly reduce their risk of developing heart disease or manage existing conditions effectively. Your heart health is in your hands, and knowledge is your greatest ally.

A heart-healthy diet is a fundamental component of reducing the risk of heart disease and maintaining cardiovascular health. The following are the key principles and fundamentals of a heart-healthy diet:

1. Limit Saturated and Trans Fats:

Saturated Fats: These fats, often found in red meat, full-fat dairy products, and some tropical oils (like coconut and palm oil), can raise LDL ("bad") cholesterol levels. Limit your intake of foods high in saturated fats.

Trans Fats: Trans fats are artificial fats created through a process called hydrogenation and are commonly found in many processed and fried foods. These fats are particularly harmful and should be avoided altogether.

2. Choose Heart-Healthy Fats:

Opt for unsaturated fats, such as monounsaturated and polyunsaturated fats, which can help lower LDL cholesterol. Good sources include olive oil, canola oil, avocados, nuts, and seeds.

3. Include Omega-3 Fatty Acids:

Omega-3 fatty acids, found in fatty fish (like salmon, mackerel, and trout), flaxseeds, chia seeds, and walnuts, can help reduce the risk of heart disease by decreasing inflammation and improving heart health.

4. Increase Fiber Intake:

Soluble fiber, found in oats, beans, fruits, and vegetables, can help lower cholesterol levels and improve heart health.

5. Consume Whole Grains:

Choose whole grains over refined grains. Whole grains like brown rice, quinoa, whole wheat pasta, and oats contain more fiber and nutrients.

6. Eat a Variety of Fruits and Vegetables:

Fruits and vegetables are rich in antioxidants, vitamins, minerals, and fiber. Aim for a colorful variety to get a wide range of nutrients.

7. Opt for Lean Proteins:

Choose lean protein sources like skinless poultry, fish, beans, lentils, tofu, and tempeh. Limit red meat consumption, and when you do eat it, choose lean cuts.

8. Control Portion Sizes:

Be mindful of portion sizes to avoid overeating and manage calorie intake.

9. Reduce Sodium Intake:

High sodium intake can lead to high blood pressure. Limit your salt intake, and use herbs, spices, and other seasonings to add flavor to your food.

10. Limit Added Sugars:

Excessive sugar consumption can contribute to obesity and heart disease. Minimize your intake of sugary snacks, desserts, and sweetened beverages.

11. Choose Low-Fat Dairy:

If you consume dairy, opt for low-fat or fat-free options to reduce saturated fat intake.

12. Stay Hydrated:

Drink plenty of water to help maintain blood volume and heart function.

13. Be Mindful of Alcohol Consumption:

If you consume alcohol, do so in moderation. Limiting alcohol intake is an important aspect of heart-healthy living.

14. Read Food Labels:

Pay attention to nutrition labels on packaged foods to make informed choices regarding their impact on heart health.

15. Plan Balanced Meals:

Create balanced meals that include a source of protein, plenty of vegetables, a whole grain, and a small amount of healthy fat.

16. Limit Processed and Fast Foods:

These foods are often high in unhealthy fats, sodium, and added sugars. Minimize their consumption.

17. Cook at Home:

Preparing your meals at home gives you more control over the ingredients and cooking methods, making it easier to follow a heart-healthy diet.

18. Be Consistent:

Consistency is key. Make these dietary changes a permanent part of your lifestyle for lasting heart health benefits.

Remember that individual dietary needs may vary, and it's essential to consult with a healthcare professional or a registered dietitian to create a personalized plan for a healthy heart, especially if you have specific dietary restrictions or health concerns. A heart-healthy diet is not only beneficial for your heart but also for your overall well-being.

COMMON HEART CONDITIONS

Heart conditions encompass a wide range of medical issues that affect the heart and its functioning. Some of the most common heart conditions include:

• Coronary Artery Disease (CAD): CAD is the most prevalent heart condition. It occurs when the coronary arteries become narrowed or blocked by the buildup of plaque, reducing blood flow to the heart muscle. This can lead to chest pain (angina) and heart attacks.

• Hypertension (High Blood Pressure): High blood pressure is a chronic condition in which the force of blood against the artery walls is consistently too high. It can lead to heart disease, stroke, and other health problems if left untreated.

• Heart Failure: Heart failure occurs when the heart can't pump blood effectively, leading to symptoms like fatigue, shortness of breath, and swelling. It can result from various heart conditions, including CAD and hypertension.

• Arrhythmias: Arrhythmias are abnormal heart rhythms. They can be too fast (tachycardia) or too slow (bradycardia) and may cause palpitations, dizziness, and fainting.

• Valvular Heart Disease: Valvular heart disease involves problems with the heart's valves, such as stenosis (narrowing) or regurgitation (leakage). These conditions can disrupt blood flow.

• Cardiomyopathy: Cardiomyopathy is a disease of the heart muscle that affects its ability to pump effectively. There are different types of cardiomyopathy, including dilated, hypertrophic, and restrictive cardiomyopathy.

• Congenital Heart Defects: Some individuals are born with structural heart abnormalities, known as congenital heart defects. These may require surgical intervention.

• Peripheral Artery Disease (PAD): PAD is a condition in which the arteries that supply blood to the extremities become narrowed or blocked, leading to reduced blood flow, particularly to the legs. It can cause leg pain and increase the risk of heart attack and stroke.

• Endocarditis: Endocarditis is an infection of the inner lining of the heart chambers and heart valves. It can be caused by bacteria entering the bloodstream and settling in the heart.

• Myocarditis: Myocarditis is inflammation of the heart muscle, often due to viral infections. It can lead to heart failure or arrhythmias.

• Pericarditis: Pericarditis is inflammation of the sac surrounding the heart (the pericardium). It can cause chest pain and discomfort.

• Aortic Aneurysm: An aortic aneurysm is a bulge or weakness in the aorta, the body's largest artery. If it ruptures, it can be life-threatening.

• Atrial Fibrillation: Atrial fibrillation (AFib) is a common arrhythmia characterized by irregular and rapid heartbeats. It can increase the risk of stroke and other heart-related complications.

• Pulmonary Hypertension: Pulmonary hypertension is high blood pressure in the arteries of the lungs, which can strain the right side of the heart.

• Rheumatic Heart Disease: This condition is a complication of untreated streptococcal infections (like strep throat) that can lead to heart valve damage.

Understanding these common heart conditions is important because it allows individuals to recognize symptoms, take preventive measures, and seek timely medical care when necessary. It's essential to consult with a healthcare professional for accurate diagnosis and appropriate treatment if you suspect any heart-related issues.

Meal planning for heart health involves making conscious choices to create balanced, nutritious meals that support cardiovascular well-being. The principles of meal planning for heart health, including portion control, are as follows:

1. Understand Nutrient Requirements:

To plan heart-healthy meals, it's essential to understand the key nutrients that promote cardiovascular health, such as fiber, healthy fats (monounsaturated and polyunsaturated fats), lean protein, and antioxidants.

2. Focus on Fiber:

Incorporate high-fiber foods like whole grains, fruits, vegetables, legumes, and nuts into your meals. Fiber helps lower cholesterol levels and maintain healthy blood pressure.

3. Choose Lean Proteins:

Opt for lean protein sources, such as skinless poultry, fish, beans, lentils, tofu, and tempeh, to reduce saturated fat intake. Limit red meat and processed meats.

4. Portion Control:

Proper portion control is crucial for maintaining a healthy weight and preventing overeating. A balanced meal should consist of:

• A serving of lean protein (about the size of your palm).

• A serving of whole grains (about half your plate).

• Plenty of vegetables (fill the remaining half of your plate).

• A small amount of healthy fat (e.g., a drizzle of olive oil or a few nuts).

• Be mindful of portion sizes when eating out, as restaurant portions can often be larger than what you need.

5. Limit Added Sugars:

Reduce the consumption of foods and beverages high in added sugars, such as sugary snacks, desserts, and sweetened beverages.

6. Control Sodium Intake:

Monitor your salt intake, as excessive sodium can lead to high blood pressure. Season food with herbs and spices instead of salt, and choose low-sodium or no-salt-added products when available.

7. Healthy Fats:

Use unsaturated fats like olive oil, avocado oil, and canola oil for cooking and as salad dressings. These fats can help improve cholesterol levels and support heart health.

8. Balanced Meals:

Create well-rounded meals that include a variety of foods from different food groups. This ensures that you get a broad range of essential nutrients.

9. Consistency:

Try to eat meals at regular intervals, as irregular eating patterns can lead to overeating or poor food choices.

10. Mindful Eating:

Pay attention to your food and savor each bite. Eating slowly and mindfully can help you recognize when you're full and prevent overeating.

11. Hydration:

Stay well-hydrated by drinking plenty of water. Proper hydration supports overall health and can help control appetite.

12. Plan Ahead:

Preparing meals in advance and having healthy snacks readily available can prevent impulsive, less healthy choices.

13. Variety:

Incorporate a wide variety of fruits, vegetables, and whole grains into your diet to ensure you receive a spectrum of essential nutrients.

14. Monitor Your Weight:

Regularly check your weight and make adjustments to your meal plan if you notice significant fluctuations.

15. Consult a Dietitian:

For personalized guidance on meal planning and portion control, consult a registered dietitian or nutritionist. They can help tailor a meal plan to your specific needs and preferences.

By following these principles of meal planning for heart health, you can create a diet that supports your cardiovascular well-being, helps maintain a healthy weight, and reduces the risk of heart disease and related complications. Remember that consistency in making these choices is key to long-term heart health.

TIPS FOR MAKING HEALTHIER CHOICES AT RESTAURANTS AND WHEN GROCERY SHOPPING

Making healthier choices at restaurants and when grocery shopping is essential for maintaining a heart-healthy diet. Here are some tips for both scenarios:

• Check the Menu in Advance: Many restaurants now provide online menus with nutritional information. Review the menu before you go to make informed choices.

• Choose Grilled or Baked Options: Opt for grilled or baked dishes rather than fried or deep-fried items, which are often higher in unhealthy fats.

• Ask for Modifications: Don't be afraid to ask for modifications to your meal, like requesting sauces on the side, substituting healthier sides (e.g., steamed vegetables instead of fries), or choosing whole-grain bread for sandwiches.

• Portion Control: Restaurant portions tend to be larger than necessary. Consider sharing an entree with a dining partner or ask for a to-go box right away to pack up half your meal.

• Select Lean Proteins: Choose dishes with lean protein sources, such as grilled chicken, fish, or legumes. Avoid dishes with fatty cuts of meat or excessive cheese.

• Avoid Sugary Drinks: Opt for water, herbal tea, or unsweetened beverages instead of sugary sodas or high-calorie cocktails.

• Ask About Sodium: If you have high blood pressure or are concerned about sodium intake, inquire about lower-sodium options and request dishes prepared with less salt.

• Mindful Eating: Eat slowly and savor each bite. This can help you recognize when you're full, preventing overeating.

When Grocery Shopping:

• Shop the Perimeter: In most grocery stores, the freshest and healthiest items like fruits, vegetables, lean meats, and dairy are usually found around the perimeter. Focus on these areas.

• Read Food Labels: Check the nutrition labels on packaged foods to evaluate the content of saturated fat, trans fat, sodium, and added sugars. Choose products with lower quantities of these components.

• Choose Whole Grains: Opt for whole-grain bread, pasta, rice, and cereals to increase your fiber intake and promote heart health.

• Select Lean Proteins: Purchase lean cuts of meat and skinless poultry. Also, consider alternative sources of protein like tofu, beans, and legumes.

• Stock Up on Fruits and Vegetables: Fill your cart with a variety of fresh, frozen, and canned fruits and vegetables. Aim for colorful options, as different colors provide different nutrients.

• Healthy Fats: Buy cooking oils like olive, canola, or avocado oil, and limit the use of butter and lard.

• Reduce Processed Foods: Minimize the number of processed and pre-packaged foods you purchase, as they often contain unhealthy additives and preservatives.

• Shop with a List: Prepare a shopping list based on your planned meals for the week. This can help you avoid impulse purchases of less healthy items.

• Don't Shop Hungry: Shopping on an empty stomach can lead to impulsive, less healthy choices. Eat a small, healthy snack before heading to the store.

• Frozen and Canned Options: Frozen and canned fruits and vegetables are convenient and can be just as nutritious as fresh options. Look for items without added sugar or salt.

• Compare Prices: Healthier options don't always have to be more expensive. Compare prices and consider buying store-brand products to save money.

• Buy in Bulk: For non-perishable items like whole grains, legumes, and canned goods, buying in bulk can be cost-effective.

By following these tips at restaurants and while grocery shopping, you can make healthier choices that support your heart health and overall well-being. Consistency in these choices is key to maintaining a heart-healthy diet.

A LIST OF HEART-HEALTHY FOODS

Heart-healthy foods are rich in nutrients that support cardiovascular health, including antioxidants, fiber, healthy fats, and various vitamins and minerals. Here's a list of heart-healthy foods to incorporate into your diet:

1. Fatty Fish:

• Salmon

• Mackerel

• Trout

• Sardines

• Herring

2. Nuts and Seeds:

• Almonds

• Walnuts

• Flaxseeds

• Chia seeds

• Pistachios

3. Berries:

• Blueberries

- Strawberries

- Raspberries

- Blackberries

4. Whole Grains:

- Oats

- Quinoa

- Brown rice

- Whole wheat pasta

- Barley

5. Leafy Greens:

- Spinach

- Kale

- Swiss chard

- Collard greens

6. Avocado

7. Legumes:

• Lentils

• Chickpeas

• Black beans

• Kidney beans

8. Tomatoes: Tomatoes are rich in lycopene, an antioxidant that supports heart health.

9. Olive Oil: Extra-virgin olive oil is a source of monounsaturated fats, which can help reduce LDL ("bad") cholesterol levels.

10. Broccoli

11. Oranges and Citrus Fruits: Oranges, grapefruits, and other citrus fruits are high in vitamin C and fiber.

12. Dark Chocolate (in moderation): Dark chocolate with a high cocoa content (70% or more) is rich in antioxidants.

13. Green Tea: Green tea is known for its high content of antioxidants and catechins, which can have a positive impact on heart health.

14. Beets

15. Pomegranates

16. Garlic: Garlic has been associated with various heart-protective benefits.

17. Red Wine (in moderation): Some studies suggest that red wine, when consumed in moderation, may have heart-protective qualities due to its resveratrol content.

18. Flaxseed Oil: Flaxseed oil is a source of omega-3 fatty acids.

19. Low-Fat Dairy: Low-fat or fat-free yogurt and milk are good sources of calcium and protein without excessive saturated fat.

20. Beans and Legumes: These are rich in fiber, protein, and various nutrients, making them excellent choices for heart health.

21. Lean Proteins: Skinless poultry, lean cuts of meat, and tofu are good sources of protein without excessive saturated fat.

22. Herbs and Spices: Herbs like rosemary, oregano, and basil, and spices like cinnamon and turmeric, have potential heart-protective properties.

Remember that while these foods can be beneficial for your heart, it's essential to maintain a balanced diet that includes a variety of nutrient-rich options and to practice portion control. Additionally, consult with a healthcare professional or a registered dietitian for personalized dietary recommendations, especially if you have specific health concerns or dietary restrictions.

NUTRITIONAL BENEFITS OF THE HEART-HEALTHY FOODS LISTED ABOVE

The heart-healthy foods listed above provide a wide array of nutritional benefits that can support cardiovascular health. Here's a breakdown of the nutritional benefits of each of these foods:

• Fatty Fish (Salmon, Mackerel, Trout, Sardines, Herring): Rich in omega-3 fatty acids, which can help reduce inflammation, lower triglycerides, and decrease the risk of heart disease.

• Nuts and Seeds (Almonds, Walnuts, Flaxseeds, Chia Seeds, Pistachios): Provide heart-healthy fats, fiber, and a variety of vitamins and minerals. They can help lower LDL cholesterol and improve overall heart health.

• Berries (Blueberries, Strawberries, Raspberries, Blackberries): Packed with antioxidants, including anthocyanins and vitamin C, which can help reduce oxidative stress and inflammation.

• Whole Grains (Oats, Quinoa, Brown Rice, Whole Wheat Pasta, Barley): High in fiber, which helps lower cholesterol levels and maintain stable blood sugar. Whole grains provide essential vitamins and minerals.

• Leafy Greens (Spinach, Kale, Swiss Chard, Collard Greens): Rich in vitamins, minerals, and fiber, they support heart health by lowering blood pressure and reducing the risk of heart disease.

• Avocado: Contains healthy monounsaturated fats, fiber, potassium, and various vitamins. Avocado can help lower bad cholesterol and reduce the risk of heart disease.

• Legumes (Lentils, Chickpeas, Black Beans, Kidney Beans): Excellent sources of fiber, protein, and essential minerals. They can help regulate blood sugar and lower LDL cholesterol.

• Tomatoes: High in lycopene, an antioxidant that may reduce the risk of heart disease by improving blood vessel function and reducing inflammation.

• Olive Oil (Extra-Virgin): Rich in monounsaturated fats and antioxidants, it can help lower LDL cholesterol and reduce the risk of heart disease.

• Broccoli: Contains fiber, vitamins, and minerals that support heart health, including antioxidants like sulforaphane.

• Oranges and Citrus Fruits: High in vitamin C, fiber, and antioxidants, they can improve blood vessel function and reduce blood pressure.

• Dark Chocolate (in moderation): Contains flavonoids, which may improve heart health by reducing inflammation and improving blood flow.

• Green Tea: Rich in antioxidants called catechins, green tea can improve cholesterol levels, reduce blood pressure, and protect the heart.

• Beets: High in dietary nitrates, which can help improve blood vessel function and lower blood pressure.

• Pomegranates: Packed with antioxidants, especially polyphenols, which can reduce inflammation and improve cholesterol profiles.

• Garlic: Contains allicin, a compound with potential heart-protective benefits, including improved cholesterol levels and reduced blood pressure.

• Red Wine (in moderation): Some studies suggest that moderate red wine consumption can raise HDL ("good") cholesterol and provide antioxidant benefits.

• Flaxseed Oil: A source of alpha-linolenic acid (ALA), a type of omega-3 fatty acid that may help reduce inflammation and lower blood pressure.

• Low-Fat Dairy: Provide essential nutrients like calcium and protein without excessive saturated fat.

• Beans and Legumes: High in fiber, protein, vitamins, and minerals. They can help regulate blood sugar and improve cholesterol levels.

• Lean Proteins: Provide essential protein without the high saturated fat content found in fatty cuts of meat.

• Herbs and Spices: Herbs and spices like rosemary, oregano, basil, cinnamon, and turmeric contain antioxidants and bioactive compounds with potential heart-protective properties.

Incorporating these heart-healthy foods into your diet can contribute to lower cholesterol, improved blood pressure, reduced inflammation, and better overall cardiovascular health. A well-rounded diet that includes a variety of these foods will provide a broad spectrum of nutrients to support your heart health.

Incorporating heart-healthy foods into your meals can be a delicious and rewarding experience. Here are some practical ways to include these foods in your diet:

1. Breakfast:

Oatmeal: Top your morning oatmeal with berries, sliced bananas, and a sprinkle of nuts or seeds for added flavor, fiber, and healthy fats.

Smoothies: Blend leafy greens, frozen berries, a ripe banana, and a tablespoon of flaxseeds or chia seeds into a nutritious and heart-healthy smoothie.

Whole Grain Cereal: Choose whole-grain cereals and add fresh fruit or a handful of nuts for extra heart-healthy goodness.

2. Snacks:

Mixed Nuts: A handful of mixed nuts, like almonds and walnuts, makes for a convenient and nutritious snack.

Greek Yogurt: Top low-fat or fat-free Greek yogurt with honey, fresh berries, and a dash of cinnamon.

Sliced Veggies: Snack on sliced cucumbers, carrots, and bell peppers with hummus for a heart-healthy crunch.

3. Lunch:

Salad: Create a colorful salad with leafy greens, cherry tomatoes, avocado, grilled chicken, and a drizzle of olive oil-based dressing.

Tuna or Salmon Sandwich: Make a tuna or salmon sandwich on whole-grain bread with plenty of fresh veggies.

Bean Soup: Enjoy a hearty bowl of bean soup, packed with fiber and protein.

4. Dinner:

Baked or Grilled Fatty Fish: Choose salmon, mackerel, or trout and serve it with a side of steamed broccoli and quinoa.

Vegetable Stir-Fry: Create a stir-fry with a variety of colorful vegetables, tofu or skinless chicken, and a sauce made with olive oil, garlic, and ginger.

Whole Wheat Pasta: Opt for whole wheat pasta and top it with a tomato-based sauce loaded with garlic, onions, and plenty of fresh basil.

5. Sides:

Sauteed Spinach: Sauté fresh spinach with a bit of olive oil and garlic for a quick and nutritious side dish.

Roasted Beets: Roast beets in the oven and serve them sliced as a side dish or in a salad.

Quinoa: Use quinoa as a side dish or as a base for grain bowls, topped with a variety of heart-healthy ingredients.

6. Desserts (in moderation):

Dark Chocolate: Savor a small piece of dark chocolate with a high cocoa content (70% or more).

Fruit Salad: Create a colorful fruit salad with a mix of berries, citrus fruits, and pomegranate seeds.

7. Beverages:

Green Tea: Enjoy green tea throughout the day. It's a heart-healthy beverage packed with antioxidants.

Smoothies: Incorporate heart-healthy ingredients like berries, flaxseeds, and spinach into your smoothies.

Remember that a balanced diet is key, so aim to create meals that include a variety of heart-healthy foods. Also, consult with a healthcare professional or a registered dietitian for personalized dietary recommendations, especially if you have specific health concerns or dietary restrictions.

COOKING METHODS THAT PROMOTE HEART HEALTH

Cooking methods that promote heart health focus on minimizing the use of unhealthy fats, reducing the formation of harmful compounds, and preserving the nutritional content of foods. Here are some cooking methods that support heart health:

1. Baking and Roasting:

Baking and roasting involve cooking food in an oven without the need for excessive added fats. They can be used for lean proteins like chicken, turkey, and fish, as well as vegetables. These methods help retain nutrients and enhance flavor.

2. Steaming:

Steaming is a heart-healthy method that uses the steam from boiling water to cook food. It preserves nutrients and flavors, especially when cooking vegetables.

3. Grilling:

Grilling, whether on a gas or charcoal grill, is a flavorful way to prepare lean meats and vegetables. It requires minimal added fats, and the fats from the food can drip away.

4. Poaching:

Poaching involves gently simmering food in water or a flavored liquid. It's a great method for cooking fish and chicken without adding extra fat.

5. Stir-Frying with Minimal Oil:

Stir-frying in a small amount of heart-healthy oil (e.g., olive oil or canola oil) can help you quickly prepare vegetables and lean proteins. Keep the oil to a minimum to limit saturated fat intake.

6. Sous Vide:

Sous vide cooking involves sealing food in a vacuum-sealed bag and cooking it in a water bath at a precise temperature. It preserves the nutrients and natural flavors of food without the need for added fats.

7. Microwaving:

Microwaving is a quick and convenient way to cook or reheat food with little to no added fat. It's an excellent method for steaming vegetables or reheating leftovers.

8. Boiling:

Boiling is suitable for foods like pasta, beans, and vegetables. To maximize nutrient retention, use as little water as necessary and avoid overcooking.

9. Herbs and Spices:

Use herbs and spices to flavor your dishes instead of excessive salt or high-sodium seasonings. This helps reduce sodium intake, which can be beneficial for heart health.

10. Reducing Frying:

Limit deep-frying or pan-frying foods in large amounts of oil, especially if the oil is high in unhealthy trans fats. If you do fry, opt for healthier oils and shallow frying with minimal oil.

11. Trimming Visible Fat:

When cooking meats, trim visible fat to reduce the saturated fat content. This can be done with poultry, beef, and pork.

12. Avoiding Processed Meats:

Minimize the consumption of processed meats like bacon, sausages, and hot dogs, which are typically high in unhealthy fats and sodium.

13. Using Non-Stick Cookware:

Non-stick cookware reduces the need for excess fats when sautéing or frying.

14. Monitoring Cooking Time:

Be mindful of cooking times to prevent overcooking, which can cause the loss of nutrients and the formation of harmful compounds.

15. Grating or Pureeing Vegetables:

Grated or pureed vegetables can be used as a healthy and flavorful base for sauces or soups, reducing the need for added fats and salt.

By using these heart-healthy cooking methods, you can enjoy delicious, nutritious meals while supporting your cardiovascular well-being. Additionally, combining these methods with a diet rich in heart-healthy ingredients can further enhance the benefits for your heart health.

DIETARY CONSIDERATIONS FOR SPECIFIC POPULATIONS, SUCH AS CHILDREN, SENIORS, OR INDIVIDUALS WITH DIETARY RESTRICTIONS (E.G., VEGETARIAN OR VEGAN).

Dietary considerations vary for specific populations, as individual nutritional needs and restrictions change with age, lifestyle, and health status. Here are some dietary considerations for different populations:

1. Children:

Nutrient-Rich Foods: Children need a variety of nutrient-rich foods to support growth and development. Include fruits, vegetables, whole grains, lean proteins, and dairy in their diets.

Calcium and Vitamin D: Ensure they get adequate calcium and vitamin D for bone health. Milk, fortified dairy alternatives, and leafy greens are good sources.

Limit Added Sugars: Minimize their intake of sugary snacks, sweetened beverages, and excessive desserts to prevent dental issues and promote healthy eating habits.

Portion Control: Serve appropriate portion sizes to avoid overeating and encourage mindful eating.

Caloric Needs: Caloric needs may decrease with age, so focus on nutrient-dense foods to meet nutritional requirements.

Protein: Seniors may need more protein to maintain muscle mass. Include lean meats, fish, beans, and dairy in their diets.

Fiber: A high-fiber diet can help prevent constipation and promote digestive health.

Vitamin B12 and Calcium: Monitor vitamin B12 intake and ensure they get enough calcium to support bone health.

Hydration: Seniors may be at risk of dehydration, so encourage them to drink water and consume hydrating foods like fruits and vegetables.

3. Individuals with Dietary Restrictions (e.g., Vegetarian or Vegan):

Protein Sources: Ensure an adequate intake of plant-based protein sources like beans, lentils, tofu, and tempeh for vegetarians and vegans.

Iron and Vitamin B12: These nutrients are often lower in plant-based diets, so incorporate iron-rich foods like spinach, fortified cereals, and foods fortified with vitamin B12.

Omega-3 Fatty Acids: Include plant-based sources of omega-3s, such as flaxseeds, chia seeds, and walnuts.

Calcium: Opt for calcium-fortified dairy alternatives like almond or soy milk.

Supplements: Depending on the diet, some individuals may require supplements for specific nutrients, especially vitamin B12 and vitamin D.

4. Individuals with Allergies or Intolerances:

Read Labels: Be vigilant about reading food labels to avoid allergens. For those with lactose intolerance, use lactose-free dairy products.

Substitutes: Identify suitable substitutes for allergenic ingredients. For example, almond milk can replace cow's milk in recipes for those with dairy allergies.

Cross-Contamination: Be aware of cross-contamination, particularly in restaurants or shared kitchen environments.

Allergen-Free Products: Utilize allergen-free products and recipes for baking and cooking.

5. Athletes:

Caloric Needs: Athletes require extra calories to fuel their activity. Focus on a balanced diet with adequate carbohydrates, proteins, and fats.

Hydration: Maintain proper hydration with water and, when necessary, sports drinks with electrolytes during intense workouts.

Recovery Foods: After exercise, consume a mix of carbohydrates and protein to aid muscle recovery.

Timing: Plan meals and snacks around training sessions to optimize energy levels and recovery.

Customizing diets to meet the unique needs and restrictions of these different populations is crucial for their health and well-being. For personalized dietary advice, consulting with a registered dietitian or healthcare professional is often beneficial to ensure that specific nutritional requirements are met.

A SHOPPING LIST FOR HEART-HEALTHY INGREDIENTS AND PANTRY STAPLES

Creating a shopping list for heart-healthy ingredients and maintaining essential pantry staples can help you consistently follow a heart-healthy diet. Here's a list of ingredients and pantry staples for your heart-healthy shopping list:

Fresh Produce:

- Leafy greens (spinach, kale, Swiss chard)

- Broccoli and cauliflower

- Tomatoes

- Bell peppers

- Carrots

- Beets

- Berries (blueberries, strawberries, raspberries)

- Citrus fruits (oranges, grapefruits, lemons)

- Avocado

- Apples

- Bananas

- Grapes

- Onions

- Garlic

- Fresh herbs (basil, rosemary, thyme)

Lean Proteins:

- Fatty fish (salmon, mackerel, trout, sardines, herring)

- Skinless poultry (chicken, turkey)

- Tofu or tempeh (for vegetarians/vegans)

- Legumes (lentils, chickpeas, black beans)

- Lean cuts of meat (if desired)

Whole Grains:

- Oats

- Quinoa

- Brown rice

- Whole wheat pasta

- Barley

Nuts and Seeds:

- Almonds

- Walnuts

- Flaxseeds

- Chia seeds

- Pistachios

Dairy and Dairy Alternatives:

- Low-fat or fat-free Greek yogurt

- Low-fat or fat-free milk

- Calcium-fortified dairy alternatives (almond, soy, or oat milk)

- Extra-virgin olive oil

- Canola oil

- Basil

- Rosemary

- Oregano

- Cinnamon

- Turmeric

- Canned tuna or salmon (in water)

- Canned beans (kidney, black, chickpeas)

- Low-sodium vegetable or chicken broth

- Whole wheat flour or almond flour

- Whole grain cereals (low in added sugars)

- Whole grain crackers

Baking Supplies:

- Whole wheat flour or almond flour

- Baking powder

- Baking soda

- Honey or maple syrup (as natural sweeteners)

Frozen Foods:

- Frozen fruits (for smoothies)

- Frozen vegetables (mixed, spinach)

- Fatty fish fillets (if fresh is not available)

Pantry Staples:

- Canned tomatoes (diced, crushed)

- Tomato paste

- Low-sodium soy sauce

- Whole grain rice or pasta

- Vinegar (balsamic, red wine)

- Whole grain or multigrain bread

- Dried herbs and spices (e.g., thyme, paprika, cumin)

Additional Pantry Items:

- Canned or dried beans (for quick protein sources)

- Low-sodium broth (vegetable, chicken)

- Whole grain crackers (for snacking)

- Nuts (store them in the pantry for easy access)

- Dried fruits (in moderation as a snack)

- Whole-grain cereal (low in added sugars)

- Natural nut butter (like almond or peanut butter)

When creating your shopping list, remember to check your pantry for any items that need restocking. Keeping these heart-healthy ingredients and pantry staples on hand will make it easier to prepare nutritious meals and snacks that support your cardiovascular health.

PRACTICAL TIPS AND TRICKS FOR MAKING HEART-HEALTHY COOKING EASY AND ENJOYABLE

Making heart-healthy cooking easy and enjoyable is all about creating a balanced approach that combines nutrition, flavor, and convenience. Here are some practical tips and tricks to help you in your heart-healthy culinary journey:

• Plan Your Meals: Spend some time each week planning your meals and snacks. This helps you make heart-healthy choices and reduce impulsive, less healthy options.

• Stock Heart-Healthy Ingredients: Keep your pantry, fridge, and freezer stocked with heart-healthy ingredients so that you can quickly put together nutritious meals.

• Prep in Advance: Prepping ingredients in advance, such as washing and chopping vegetables, can save time and make cooking less daunting.

• Experiment with Herbs and Spices: Herbs and spices are your friends for adding flavor without relying on salt. Get creative with seasonings to keep your meals interesting.

• Use Healthy Cooking Oils: Opt for heart-healthy oils like extra-virgin olive oil or canola oil for cooking and salad dressings.

• Control Portions: Be mindful of portion sizes. Use smaller plates and utensils to help with portion control.

• Balance Your Plate: Aim to fill half your plate with vegetables, a quarter with lean protein, and a quarter with whole grains. This creates a balanced meal.

• Learn Cooking Techniques: Invest time in learning basic cooking techniques such as roasting, grilling, and steaming to make healthier meals.

• Cook with Lean Proteins: Use lean cuts of meat and skinless poultry, or opt for plant-based protein sources like tofu and legumes.

• Include Fatty Fish: Incorporate fatty fish like salmon into your diet at least twice a week to benefit from omega-3 fatty acids.

• Experiment with Plant-Based Meals: Try vegetarian or vegan recipes to reduce saturated fat intake and increase your intake of fruits, vegetables, and legumes.

• Hydrate Wisely: Drink plenty of water throughout the day. Staying well-hydrated is essential for overall health and appetite control.

• Moderate Your Sweet Tooth: Reduce your consumption of sugary snacks, desserts, and sugary beverages. Opt for healthier alternatives like fresh fruit or yogurt with honey.

• Minimize Processed Foods: Limit the consumption of highly processed and packaged foods, which often contain unhealthy additives and preservatives.

• Keep Healthy Snacks Ready: Have a supply of healthy snacks like cut vegetables, whole fruit, nuts, or yogurt on hand for quick, satisfying nibbles.

• Set Realistic Goals: Don't feel pressured to make drastic changes overnight. Small, sustainable changes can lead to long-term success.

• Cook with Family and Friends: Involve family members or friends in cooking. It can be a fun and social activity that helps build support for your heart-healthy goals.

• Celebrate Diversity: Explore diverse cuisines and try new ingredients to keep your meals interesting and exciting.

• Listen to Your Body: Pay attention to your body's hunger and fullness cues. Eating mindfully can help prevent overeating.

• Seek Support: Join a heart-healthy cooking group or follow online resources and blogs for inspiration and guidance.

Remember that creating a heart-healthy diet is a journey, not a destination. Be patient with yourself, enjoy the process, and savor the delicious, nutritious meals you prepare.

THE IMPORTANCE OF REGULAR EXERCISE, STRESS MANAGEMENT, AND GETTING ADEQUATE SLEEP IN ADDITION TO HEALTHY EATING FOR OVERALL HEART HEALTH.

Heart health is not solely about what you eat; it's a multifaceted approach that includes various lifestyle factors. In addition to a healthy diet, regular exercise, stress management, and adequate sleep are crucial components for overall heart health. Here's why each of these factors is important:

1. Regular Exercise: Exercise is a cornerstone of heart health for several reasons:

• Strengthening the Heart: Regular physical activity makes your heart stronger, enabling it to pump blood more efficiently and reducing the workload on the heart.

• Improving Cholesterol Profiles: Exercise helps raise HDL ("good") cholesterol and lower LDL ("bad") cholesterol levels, reducing the risk of plaque buildup in your arteries.

• Controlling Blood Pressure: Physical activity can help lower high blood pressure, which is a major risk factor for heart disease.

• Enhancing Blood Sugar Control: Exercise aids in regulating blood sugar levels, reducing the risk of diabetes, which is a significant contributor to heart disease.

• Aiding in Weight Management: Physical activity helps with weight loss and maintenance, which is vital for heart health as excess body weight increases the risk of heart disease.

• Enhancing Circulation: Exercise promotes healthy blood vessel function, reducing the risk of blood clots and improving overall circulation.

2. Stress Management: Chronic stress can have a detrimental impact on heart health:

• High Blood Pressure: Stress triggers the release of stress hormones, which can raise blood pressure, putting extra strain on the heart.

• Inflammation: Long-term stress can lead to chronic inflammation, which is a risk factor for heart disease.

• Unhealthy Coping Mechanisms: Some people cope with stress through unhealthy habits like overeating, smoking, or excessive alcohol consumption, which can harm the heart.

• Poor Sleep: Stress can lead to poor sleep quality, and inadequate sleep is associated with an increased risk of heart disease.

Effective stress management techniques, such as meditation, deep breathing, yoga, and regular physical activity, can help reduce stress and its impact on the heart.

3. Adequate Sleep: Sleep is a critical component of heart health:

• Rest and Repair: During sleep, the body repairs and regenerates tissues, including the heart and blood vessels.

• Hormonal Balance: Sleep helps regulate hormones that affect appetite, metabolism, and stress, all of which can impact heart health.

• Blood Pressure Control: Adequate sleep plays a role in keeping blood pressure in check.

• Weight Management: Lack of sleep can disrupt hormones that control hunger and appetite, leading to weight gain.

• Cognitive Function: Poor sleep can affect cognitive function, which can impact decisions related to diet and exercise.

• To support heart health, aim for 7-9 hours of quality sleep each night.

In summary, a heart-healthy lifestyle involves a holistic approach. Eating a nutritious diet is a foundational aspect, but it must be combined with regular exercise, effective stress management, and adequate sleep to achieve optimal cardiovascular well-being. It's essential to embrace these lifestyle choices collectively to reduce the risk of heart disease and improve overall quality of life.

THE IMPORTANCE OF MODERATION AND BALANCE IN ALL ASPECTS OF DIET AND LIFESTYLE.

Moderation and balance are fundamental principles of maintaining a healthy and sustainable lifestyle, especially when it comes to diet and overall well-being. Here's why they are essential:

1. Diet:

• Nutritional Balance: A balanced diet includes a variety of foods from all food groups, providing essential nutrients. It allows you to meet your nutritional needs, supporting overall health and preventing deficiencies.

• Portion Control: Moderation in portion sizes helps you manage your calorie intake, promoting a healthy weight. Overeating, even healthy foods, can lead to weight gain and associated health risks.

• Diverse Food Choices: A balanced diet encourages the consumption of a wide range of foods, ensuring you benefit from various vitamins, minerals, and antioxidants. Over-reliance on a limited set of foods may lead to nutrient imbalances.

• Preventing Overindulgence: Consuming treats and indulgent foods in moderation allows you to enjoy them without overloading your body with excess sugar, unhealthy fats, or sodium.

• Avoiding Extreme Diets: Extreme dieting can be harmful and unsustainable. Strive for balance by avoiding restrictive diets and finding a reasonable approach to eating that suits your needs.

2. Physical Activity:

• Avoiding Overtraining: Balance in exercise prevents overtraining and the risk of injury. Rest and recovery are as crucial as active workouts to support long-term fitness and health goals.

• Adaptation: Regular, balanced exercise helps your body adapt to increased demands over time, promoting overall physical well-being without overexertion.

• Incorporating Variety: Balance your fitness routine by incorporating a mix of cardiovascular, strength, and flexibility exercises. This provides holistic benefits for your body.

3. Stress Management:

• Preventing Burnout: Balancing work, family, and personal time is essential to prevent burnout and chronic stress. Chronic stress can lead to physical and mental health issues, including heart problems.

• Mental Health: Balance in stress management techniques, such as relaxation, mindfulness, and time for self-care, supports your mental health and emotional well-being.

4. Sleep:

• Prioritizing Sleep: Adequate sleep is essential for physical and mental recovery. Balancing your schedule to ensure you get enough rest supports cognitive function, emotional stability, and overall health.

• Avoiding Excess: Overindulging in sleep (oversleeping) can also have adverse effects on your health, so finding the right balance is crucial.

5. Social and Personal Life:

• Balancing Social and Personal Needs: Maintaining a healthy social life while nurturing personal well-being is essential. It prevents isolation and supports emotional health.

• Managing Commitments: Balancing commitments to work, family, and personal interests helps you avoid excessive stress and burnout.

6. Financial Health:

• Budgeting: Financial balance involves budgeting, saving, and managing expenses. It ensures you don't overspend, leading to financial stress.

• Investing: Balanced financial planning includes investments to secure your future while enjoying your present.

In conclusion, moderation and balance in all aspects of diet and lifestyle are vital for long-term health, well-being, and happiness. By adopting a balanced approach, you can enjoy the pleasures of life without overindulging, maintain a sustainable and healthy routine, and reduce the risk of negative health outcomes. Achieving this equilibrium is a continuous journey that requires self-awareness and conscious decision-making to support your overall heart health and quality of life.

HOW TO READ AND INTERPRET NUTRITION LABELS TO MAKE INFORMED FOOD CHOICES

Reading and interpreting nutrition labels is a valuable skill that allows you to make informed food choices and support your overall health and dietary goals. Here's a step-by-step guide on how to read and understand nutrition labels:

1. Start with the Serving Size: The serving size is listed at the top of the nutrition label. All the information on the label is based on this serving size, so make sure to compare it to the portion you intend to eat.

2. Check the Calories: The number of calories per serving indicates how much energy you will get from that portion. Be mindful of portion size, as it affects the total calorie intake.

3. Examine Macronutrients: Look at the total amounts of macronutrients per serving:

• Total Fat: Pay attention to the amount of saturated and trans fats. Limit saturated and trans fats, as they can raise LDL cholesterol (the "bad" cholesterol).

• Cholesterol: High cholesterol intake can also contribute to heart disease. Aim to consume less than 300 milligrams per day.

• Sodium: Excessive sodium intake can increase blood pressure. The recommended daily sodium intake is typically less than 2,300 milligrams.

• Total Carbohydrates: Consider the amount of dietary fiber (good) and added sugars (limit added sugars as they provide extra calories with few nutrients).

• Protein: Ensure you get enough protein, but don't overconsume, as excessive protein can be stored as fat.

4. Fiber and Sugars: Pay attention to dietary fiber and added sugars. A high-fiber diet supports digestive health, while excessive added sugars can lead to weight gain and health issues.

5. Micronutrients: Check the percentages of vitamins and minerals like vitamin D, calcium, iron, and potassium. A label may also indicate if the food is a good source of a particular nutrient.

6. Percent Daily Value (%DV): %DV helps you understand how the nutrients in one serving fit into your daily diet. As a general rule, aim for nutrients with a %DV of 5% or less (low) and nutrients with a %DV of 20% or more (high).

7. Ingredients List: Scan the list of ingredients. Ingredients are listed in order of highest quantity to lowest. Be wary of foods with long lists of artificial additives and preservatives.

8. Allergen Information: Check for allergen warnings, especially if you have food allergies or intolerances. Labels typically list common allergens like peanuts, tree nuts, soy, dairy, and wheat.

9. Health Claims: Be cautious of health claims on food packaging, as they can sometimes be misleading. Focus on the nutrition label and ingredient list for accurate information.

10. Compare Similar Products: When shopping, compare the nutrition labels of similar products to make the healthiest choice. Pay attention to serving size when comparing.

11. Context Matters: Consider the context of your overall diet and health goals. What may be considered "good" or "bad" on a nutrition label depends on your individual dietary needs.

Remember that interpreting nutrition labels is a valuable tool for making informed food choices, but it's just one aspect of maintaining a balanced and healthy diet. Consider consulting with a registered dietitian for personalized guidance based on your specific dietary requirements and health goals.

HOW TO REPLACE OR REDUCE UNHEALTHY FATS IN RECIPES

Replacing or reducing unhealthy fats in recipes is a great way to make your meals and dishes more heart-healthy. Unhealthy fats, such as saturated and trans fats, can contribute to high cholesterol and heart disease. Here are some tips on how to replace or reduce these fats in your cooking:

• Use Healthier Cooking Oils: Replace butter and lard with healthier oils like olive oil, canola oil, or avocado oil. These oils are high in monounsaturated and polyunsaturated fats, which are better for your heart.

• Opt for Non-Stick Cookware: Non-stick pans and cooking sprays allow you to use less oil when cooking without the risk of sticking.

• Choose Lean Cuts of Meat: Select lean cuts of meat, trim visible fat, and remove the skin from poultry. This reduces saturated fat content in your dishes.

• Incorporate Plant-Based Proteins: Replace some or all of the meat in your recipes with plant-based protein sources like tofu, tempeh, beans, lentils, and legumes, which are naturally low in unhealthy fats.

• Use Low-Fat Dairy or Dairy Alternatives: Substitute whole-fat dairy products with low-fat or fat-free options. For dairy alternatives, choose unsweetened versions for recipes that call for milk or yogurt.

• Avocado as a Butter Substitute: In baking, replace some or all of the butter in recipes with mashed avocado. This adds healthy fats and moisture.

• Nut and Seed Butters: Use nut and seed butters (e.g., almond butter, peanut butter, or tahini) as spreads or in recipes instead of butter or cream cheese. They provide heart-healthy fats.

• Add Pureed Fruits and Vegetables: In baking, consider adding pureed fruits or vegetables (like applesauce, mashed bananas, or pureed sweet potatoes) to replace some of the fat. This can add moisture and flavor.

• Choose Reduced-Fat Ingredients: Select reduced-fat or fat-free versions of mayonnaise, salad dressings, and condiments. These options often contain less unhealthy fat.

• Limit Fried Foods: Avoid deep-frying your foods. Instead, use healthier cooking methods like baking, grilling, or steaming.

• Roasting and Grilling: Roasting or grilling can add flavor and texture to dishes without the need for excessive fats.

• Use Fresh Herbs and Spices: Experiment with herbs and spices to add flavor without relying on excess salt or fats.

• Homemade Sauces and Dressings: Make your own sauces and salad dressings using healthier oils, herbs, and spices. This way, you can control the fat content.

• Cook with Broths and Stocks: Use vegetable or chicken broth for sautéing and cooking instead of butter or oil.

• Read Food Labels: When purchasing pre-packaged foods or condiments, check the labels for saturated and trans fats. Choose products with lower amounts of these unhealthy fats.

Remember that small changes in your cooking and ingredient choices can add up to significant reductions in unhealthy fats in your diet. Focus on cooking methods and ingredients that promote heart health and enjoy delicious, heart-healthy meals.

CHAPTER TWO

BREAKFAST RECIPES

Oatmeal with Berries and Nuts

Ingredients:

• 1/2 cup old-fashioned oats

• 1 cup low-fat milk or a dairy-free alternative

• 1/2 cup mixed berries (blueberries, strawberries, raspberries)

• 1 tablespoon chopped nuts (almonds, walnuts)

• 1 teaspoon honey or pure maple syrup (optional)

• A dash of cinnamon

Instructions:

1. In a saucepan, combine the oats and milk. Cook over medium heat, stirring occasionally until the oats are creamy and cooked to your desired consistency.

2. Pour the oatmeal into a bowl and top with mixed berries, chopped nuts, a drizzle of honey or maple syrup (if desired), and a dash of cinnamon.

Greek Yogurt Parfait

Ingredients:

• 1 cup low-fat Greek yogurt

• 1/2 cup mixed berries

• 1 tablespoon honey or pure maple syrup

• 1/4 cup granola

• 1 teaspoon chia seeds (optional)

Instructions:

1. In a glass or bowl, layer the Greek yogurt, mixed berries, and granola.

2. Drizzle honey or maple syrup over the top and sprinkle with chia seeds, if desired.

Ingredients:

• 1 whole-grain toast

• 1/2 ripe avocado, mashed

• Sliced tomatoes

• Salt and pepper to taste

• Optional toppings: a sprinkle of feta cheese, red pepper flakes, or fresh herbs

Instructions:

1. Toast the whole-grain bread.

2. Spread the mashed avocado on the toast and top with sliced tomatoes.

3. Season with a pinch of salt and pepper. Add optional toppings like crumbled feta cheese, red pepper flakes, or fresh herbs for extra flavor.

Ingredients:

• 2 egg whites

• Handful of spinach leaves

• Sliced mushrooms

• Chopped bell peppers (optional)

• Chopped onion (optional)

• Salt and pepper to taste

• Olive oil or cooking spray

Instructions:

1. Heat a non-stick skillet over medium heat and lightly coat it with olive oil or cooking spray.

2. Sauté the mushrooms (and other veggies, if using) until they start to soften.

3. Add the spinach and cook until wilted. Pour the egg whites over the veggies and cook until set, folding it in half like an omelette.

4. Season with salt and pepper and serve.

Chia Seed Pudding

Ingredients:

• 2 tablespoons chia seeds

• 1/2 cup almond milk (or your choice of milk)

• 1/2 teaspoon vanilla extract

• Sliced fresh fruit (e.g., bananas, strawberries, or kiwi)

• A drizzle of honey or pure maple syrup (optional)

Instructions:

1. In a bowl, combine the chia seeds, almond milk, and vanilla extract. Stir well.

2. Cover the bowl and refrigerate for at least a few hours or overnight to allow the chia seeds to absorb the liquid and create a pudding-like consistency.

3. Before serving, top the chia seed pudding with sliced fresh fruit and a drizzle of honey or maple syrup if you prefer a touch of sweetness.

Whole Grain Pancakes with Fruit

Ingredients:

• 1/2 cup whole wheat flour

• 1/4 cup rolled oats

• 1/2 teaspoon baking powder

• 1/2 cup low-fat milk or dairy-free alternative

• 1 egg (or flaxseed egg for a vegan option)

• 1/2 teaspoon vanilla extract

• Sliced bananas, berries, or apples

• Greek yogurt or a dairy-free alternative

• Pure maple syrup (in moderation)

Instructions:

1. In a mixing bowl, combine the whole wheat flour, rolled oats, and baking powder.

2. Add milk, egg, and vanilla extract, and stir until well mixed.

3. Heat a non-stick skillet and ladle the pancake batter onto it. Cook until bubbles form, then flip and cook until golden.

4. Serve pancakes with a dollop of Greek yogurt and your choice of fresh fruit. Drizzle with a touch of pure maple syrup if desired.

Veggie and Egg Breakfast Burrito

Ingredients:

• Whole-grain tortilla

• 2 egg whites

• Sliced bell peppers, onions, and tomatoes

• Spinach leaves

• Salsa or hot sauce (for added flavor)

• A sprinkle of reduced-fat cheese (optional)

Instructions:

1. In a non-stick skillet, sauté the sliced veggies until they're tender and slightly caramelized.

2. Add the egg whites and scramble them with the veggies.

3. Place the veggie and egg mixture onto a whole-grain tortilla.

4. Top with fresh spinach leaves, salsa or hot sauce, and a sprinkle of reduced-fat cheese, if desired. Roll it up and enjoy.

Quinoa Breakfast Bowl

Ingredients:

• Cooked quinoa

• Sliced fresh fruit (e.g., mango, strawberries, or kiwi)

• Chopped nuts (e.g., almonds or walnuts)

• A drizzle of honey or pure maple syrup (optional)

Instructions:

1. In a bowl, place a serving of cooked quinoa.

2. Top with sliced fresh fruit and chopped nuts.

3. Drizzle with a small amount of honey or maple syrup for a touch of sweetness.

Spinach and Mushroom Breakfast Quesadilla

Ingredients:

• Whole-grain tortilla

• Handful of spinach leaves

• Sliced mushrooms

• Sliced bell peppers (optional)

• Reduced-fat cheese

• A sprinkle of your favorite herbs and spices

Instructions:

1. In a non-stick skillet, sauté the mushrooms (and bell peppers if using) until tender.

2. Place a whole-grain tortilla in the skillet.

3. Layer with spinach leaves, sautéed mushrooms, and reduced-fat cheese.

4. Top with another tortilla and cook until the cheese melts and the tortilla is golden brown. Slice and enjoy.

Peanut Butter and Banana Toast

Ingredients:

• Whole-grain toast

• Natural peanut butter (or almond butter)

• Sliced bananas

• A sprinkle of chia seeds (optional)

Instructions:

1. Toast a slice of whole-grain bread.

2. Spread a thin layer of natural peanut butter on the toast.

3. Top with sliced bananas and a sprinkle of chia seeds for added crunch and nutrition.

Berry and Greek Yogurt Smoothie

Ingredients:

• 1 cup low-fat Greek yogurt

• 1/2 cup mixed berries (strawberries, blueberries, raspberries)

• 1 ripe banana

• 1 tablespoon honey or pure maple syrup (optional)

• 1/4 cup rolled oats

• Ice cubes (if desired)

Instructions:

1. Blend Greek yogurt, mixed berries, banana, and honey or maple syrup until smooth.

2. Add rolled oats and blend again until well combined.

3. If you prefer a colder texture, add a few ice cubes and blend until smooth.

Ingredients:

• 2 eggs

• Sliced cherry tomatoes

• Chopped spinach

• Chopped bell peppers (optional)

• Crumbled feta cheese

• Fresh herbs (e.g., basil, chives, or parsley)

• Salt and pepper to taste

• Cooking spray or a small amount of olive oil

Instructions:

1. Heat a non-stick skillet and coat it with cooking spray or a small amount of olive oil.

2. In a bowl, whisk the eggs, salt, and pepper. Pour the egg mixture into the skillet.

3. Add the sliced tomatoes, chopped spinach, and bell peppers. Cook until the eggs are set but still moist.

4. Sprinkle crumbled feta cheese and fresh herbs on top. Serve hot.

Whole Grain Cereal with Fresh Fruit

Ingredients:

• Whole-grain cereal (e.g., bran flakes, whole grain oats)

• Low-fat milk or dairy-free alternative

• Sliced fresh fruit (e.g., peaches, strawberries, or kiwi)

• A sprinkle of ground flaxseed (optional)

• A dash of cinnamon

Instructions:

1. Pour whole-grain cereal into a bowl.

2. Add low-fat milk or a dairy-free alternative. Top with sliced fresh fruit.

3. Sprinkle ground flaxseed and a dash of cinnamon for added flavor and fiber.

Sweet Potato and Black Bean Breakfast Burrito

Ingredients:

• Whole-grain tortilla

• Scrambled eggs (or tofu scramble for a vegan option)

• Roasted sweet potato cubes

• Black beans (canned, drained and rinsed)

• Salsa or hot sauce (for added flavor)

• Avocado slices

Instructions:

1. Fill a whole-grain tortilla with scrambled eggs (or tofu scramble), roasted sweet potato cubes, and black beans.

2. Top with salsa or hot sauce and avocado slices.

3. Roll it up and enjoy your heart-healthy breakfast burrito.

Green Smoothie Bowl

Ingredients:

• 1 cup spinach or kale leaves

• 1/2 frozen banana

• 1/2 cup low-fat Greek yogurt or dairy-free alternative

• 1/4 cup unsweetened almond milk (or your choice of milk)

• Toppings: sliced kiwi, shredded coconut, chia seeds, and a drizzle of honey

Instructions:

1. Blend spinach or kale, frozen banana, Greek yogurt, and almond milk until smooth.

2. Pour the green smoothie into a bowl.

3. Top with sliced kiwi, shredded coconut, chia seeds, and a drizzle of honey.

Chia Seed and Fruit Pudding

Ingredients:

- 2 tablespoons chia seeds

- 1/2 cup low-fat milk or dairy-free alternative

- 1/2 teaspoon vanilla extract

- Sliced fresh fruit (e.g., strawberries, blueberries, or mango)

- A drizzle of honey or pure maple syrup (optional)

Instructions:

1. In a jar or bowl, mix chia seeds, milk, and vanilla extract.

2. Stir well, cover, and refrigerate for a few hours or overnight until it thickens to a pudding-like consistency.

3. Top with sliced fresh fruit and a drizzle of honey or maple syrup if desired.

Whole Grain Breakfast Burrito

Ingredients:

- Whole-grain tortilla

- Scrambled eggs (or tofu scramble for a vegan option)

- Sliced avocado

- Salsa or hot sauce (for added flavor)

- Fresh cilantro leaves

Instructions:

1. Fill a whole-grain tortilla with scrambled eggs (or tofu scramble), sliced avocado, salsa or hot sauce, and fresh cilantro leaves.

2. Roll it up and enjoy your heart-healthy breakfast burrito.

Overnight Oats with Almonds and Berries

Ingredients:

- 1/2 cup rolled oats

- 1/2 cup low-fat milk or dairy-free alternative

- Sliced almonds

- Mixed berries (e.g., raspberries, blackberries)

- A drizzle of honey or pure maple syrup (optional)

Instructions:

1. In a jar or container, combine rolled oats and milk.

2. Stir, cover, and refrigerate overnight.

3. In the morning, top with sliced almonds, mixed berries, and a drizzle of honey or maple syrup if desired.

Peanut Butter and Chia Toast

Ingredients:

• Whole-grain toast

• Natural peanut butter (or almond butter)

• Sliced banana

• Chia seeds

Instructions:

1. Toast a slice of whole-grain bread.

2. Spread a thin layer of natural peanut butter on the toast.

3. Top with sliced banana and a sprinkle of chia seeds.

Ingredients:

• 2 eggs

• Chopped bell peppers, onions, and tomatoes

• Chopped fresh herbs (e.g., basil, chives, or parsley)

• Salt and pepper to taste

• Cooking spray or a small amount of olive oil

Instructions:

1. Heat a non-stick skillet and coat it with cooking spray or a small amount of olive oil.

2. In a bowl, whisk the eggs, salt, and pepper. Pour the egg mixture into the skillet.

3. Add the chopped bell peppers, onions, and tomatoes. Cook until the eggs are set but still moist.

4. Sprinkle chopped fresh herbs on top and serve hot.

Ingredients:

• Whole-grain toast

• 1 ripe avocado, mashed

• Sliced tomatoes

• Fresh basil leaves

• Salt and pepper to taste

• A drizzle of balsamic vinegar (optional)

Instructions:

1. Toast a slice of whole-grain bread.

2. Spread the mashed avocado on the toast. Top with sliced tomatoes and fresh basil leaves.

3. Season with salt and pepper, and add a drizzle of balsamic vinegar for extra flavor.

Berry and Almond Butter Smoothie

Ingredients:

• 1 cup unsweetened almond milk (or your choice of milk)

• 1/2 banana

• 1/2 cup mixed berries (e.g., blueberries, raspberries, strawberries)

• 1 tablespoon almond butter

• 1/4 cup plain low-fat Greek yogurt (or dairy-free alternative)

• A drizzle of honey (optional)

Instructions:

1. Blend almond milk, banana, mixed berries, almond butter, Greek yogurt, and honey until smooth.

2. Pour into a glass and enjoy this heart-healthy smoothie.

Spinach and Feta Breakfast Wrap

Ingredients:

• Whole-grain tortilla

• Scrambled eggs (or tofu scramble for a vegan option)

- Sautéed spinach

- Crumbled feta cheese

- Fresh dill (optional)

- Salsa (for added flavor)

Instructions:

1. Fill a whole-grain tortilla with scrambled eggs (or tofu scramble), sautéed spinach, crumbled feta cheese, and fresh dill.

2. Top with salsa for an extra burst of flavor.

Peanut Butter and Banana Overnight Oats

Ingredients:

- 1/2 cup rolled oats

- 1/2 cup low-fat milk or dairy-free alternative

- 2 tablespoons natural peanut butter (or almond butter)

- 1 ripe banana, sliced

- A dash of cinnamon

- A sprinkle of chopped nuts (e.g., almonds or walnuts)

Instructions:

1. In a jar or container, combine rolled oats, milk, peanut butter, and a dash of cinnamon.

2. Stir well, cover, and refrigerate overnight.

3. In the morning, top with sliced banana and a sprinkle of chopped nuts.

Mediterranean Breakfast Bowl

Ingredients:

- Cooked quinoa

- Sliced cucumber

- Cherry tomatoes, halved

- Kalamata olives, pitted and sliced

- Feta cheese

• Fresh parsley

• Olive oil and lemon juice for dressing

Instructions:

1. In a bowl, place a serving of cooked quinoa.

2. Top with sliced cucumber, halved cherry tomatoes, sliced Kalamata olives, and crumbled feta cheese.

3. Drizzle with a dressing made from olive oil and lemon juice.

4. Garnish with fresh parsley.

Grilled Salmon Salad

Ingredients:

• 6-8 ounces of grilled salmon (seasoned with herbs and lemon)

• Mixed salad greens (e.g., spinach, arugula, and romaine)

• Cherry tomatoes

• Cucumber slices

• Red onion, thinly sliced

• Avocado slices

• Balsamic vinaigrette dressing (choose a low-sodium option)

Instructions:

1. Grill the salmon with herbs and lemon until it flakes easily.

2. On a plate, arrange the mixed salad greens, cherry tomatoes, cucumber, red onion, and avocado.

3. Top the salad with the grilled salmon and drizzle with balsamic vinaigrette.

Ingredients:

• 1 cup cooked quinoa

• Mixed vegetables (e.g., bell peppers, broccoli, carrots, snap peas)

• Low-sodium soy sauce or tamari

• Garlic and ginger for flavor

• Chopped green onions

• Sesame seeds

Instructions:

1. In a wok or large skillet, stir-fry mixed vegetables with garlic and ginger until tender.

2. Add cooked quinoa and low-sodium soy sauce or tamari. Stir to combine.

3. Serve the stir-fry with a sprinkle of chopped green onions and sesame seeds.

Ingredients:

• Whole-grain wrap or tortilla

• Mashed avocado

• Canned chickpeas, drained and rinsed

• Sliced red onion

• Spinach leaves

• Sliced red bell pepper

• Hummus (as a spread)

• A squeeze of lemon juice

• Salt and pepper to taste

Instructions:

1. Spread mashed avocado and hummus on the whole-grain wrap.

2. Top with chickpeas, red onion, spinach, and red bell pepper. Drizzle with lemon juice and season with salt and pepper.

3. Roll up the wrap and enjoy.

Lentil and Vegetable Soup

Ingredients:

• 1 cup dried green or brown lentils (rinsed)

• Mixed vegetables (e.g., carrots, celery, zucchini)

• Onion and garlic, chopped

• Low-sodium vegetable broth

• Fresh herbs (e.g., thyme and rosemary)

• Salt and pepper to taste

Instructions:

1. In a large pot, sauté onions, garlic, and mixed vegetables until they soften.

2. Add dried lentils and cover with low-sodium vegetable broth. Season with fresh herbs, salt, and pepper.

3. Simmer until the lentils are tender and the soup is flavorful.

Ingredients:

• Sliced turkey breast (low-sodium, nitrate-free)

• Mixed salad greens

• Sliced avocado

• Cherry tomatoes

• Cucumber slices

• Light vinaigrette dressing (choose a low-sodium option)

Instructions:

1. On a plate, arrange mixed salad greens, cherry tomatoes, cucumber, and sliced avocado.

2. Top with sliced turkey breast.

3. Drizzle with a light vinaigrette dressing.

Ingredients:

• 1 cup cooked quinoa

• 1 can black beans, drained and rinsed

• Red bell pepper, diced

• Corn kernels (fresh or frozen)

• Red onion, finely chopped

• Fresh cilantro, chopped

• Lime juice

• Olive oil

• Salt and pepper to taste

Instructions:

1. In a large bowl, combine cooked quinoa, black beans, red bell pepper, corn, and red onion.

2. Drizzle with a dressing made from fresh cilantro, lime juice, olive oil, salt, and pepper.

3. Toss to combine and enjoy this hearty and flavorful salad.

Grilled Chicken and Vegetable Wrap

Ingredients:

• Grilled chicken breast, sliced

• Whole-grain wrap or tortilla

• Hummus

• Sliced cucumber

• Sliced red bell pepper

• Spinach leaves

• A squeeze of lemon juice

• Salt and pepper to taste

Instructions:

1. Spread a layer of hummus on the whole-grain wrap.

2. Top with sliced grilled chicken, cucumber, red bell pepper, and spinach. Drizzle with lemon juice and season with salt and pepper.

3. Roll up the wrap for a satisfying and heart-healthy lunch.

Tomato and Basil Quinoa Salad

Ingredients:

• 1 cup cooked quinoa

• Fresh tomatoes, diced

• Fresh basil leaves, chopped

• Red onion, finely chopped

• Balsamic vinegar

• Olive oil

• Salt and pepper to taste

Instructions:

1. In a bowl, combine cooked quinoa, diced tomatoes, chopped basil, and finely chopped red onion.

2. Drizzle with balsamic vinegar and olive oil, and season with salt and pepper.

3. Toss to combine, and enjoy this light and flavorful quinoa salad.

Veggie and Lentil Soup

Ingredients:

- 1 cup dried green or brown lentils (rinsed)

- Mixed vegetables (e.g., carrots, celery, spinach)

- Onion and garlic, chopped

- Low-sodium vegetable broth

- Fresh thyme and bay leaves

- Salt and pepper to taste

Instructions:

1. In a large pot, sauté onions, garlic, and mixed vegetables until they soften.

2. Add dried lentils and cover with low-sodium vegetable broth. Add fresh thyme and bay leaves, and season with salt and pepper.

3. Simmer until the lentils are tender and the soup is full of flavor.

Mediterranean Hummus Bowl

Ingredients:

• Hummus (choose your favorite flavor)

• Cherry tomatoes, halved

• Cucumber slices

• Kalamata olives, pitted and sliced

• Feta cheese (choose a reduced-fat option)

• Fresh parsley

• Whole-grain pita or flatbread

Instructions:

1. In a bowl, spread a generous portion of hummus as the base.

2. Top with cherry tomatoes, cucumber slices, Kalamata olives, and crumbled feta cheese. Garnish with fresh parsley.

3. Serve with whole-grain pita or flatbread for dipping.

Chickpea and Spinach Salad

Ingredients:

• 1 can chickpeas, drained and rinsed

• Fresh baby spinach

• Cherry tomatoes, halved

• Red onion, thinly sliced

• Feta cheese (choose a reduced-fat option)

• Balsamic vinaigrette dressing (choose a low-sodium option)

Instructions:

1. In a large bowl, combine chickpeas, fresh baby spinach, cherry tomatoes, red onion, and crumbled feta cheese.

2. Drizzle with balsamic vinaigrette dressing and toss to coat.

Ingredients:

• Canned tuna in water, drained

• Canned white beans, drained and rinsed

• Red onion, finely chopped

• Chopped celery

• Fresh parsley, chopped

• Lemon juice

• Olive oil

• Salt and pepper to taste

Instructions:

1. In a bowl, combine canned tuna, white beans, red onion, chopped celery, and fresh parsley.

2. Drizzle with lemon juice and olive oil, and season with salt and pepper.

3. Toss to combine and enjoy this protein-packed salad.

Whole Grain Pita with Hummus and Veggies

Ingredients:

• Whole grain pita bread

• Hummus (choose your favorite flavor)

• Sliced cucumbers

• Sliced red bell pepper

• Cherry tomatoes, halved

• Baby carrots

• Sliced radishes

Instructions:

1. Cut the whole grain pita bread into halves.

2. Spread hummus on the pita halves.

3. Top with sliced cucumbers, red bell pepper, cherry tomatoes, baby carrots, and sliced radishes.

Ingredients:

• Grilled mixed vegetables (e.g., zucchini, bell peppers, asparagus)

• Cooked quinoa

• Cherry tomatoes

• Fresh basil leaves

• Balsamic vinegar and olive oil

• Salt and pepper to taste

Instructions:

1. Arrange grilled mixed vegetables on a plate or in a bowl.

2. Add cooked quinoa and cherry tomatoes. Drizzle with balsamic vinegar and olive oil.

3. Season with salt and pepper and garnish with fresh basil leaves.

Ingredients:

• Boneless, skinless chicken breast, sliced

• Mixed vegetables (e.g., broccoli, bell peppers, snap peas)

• Garlic and ginger for flavor

• Low-sodium soy sauce or tamari

• Cooked brown rice

Instructions:

1. In a wok or large skillet, stir-fry chicken with garlic and ginger until cooked through.

2. Add mixed vegetables and continue stir-frying until they are tender. Add low-sodium soy sauce or tamari for flavor.

3. Serve over cooked brown rice for a satisfying stir-fry.

Spinach and Strawberry Salad with Grilled Chicken

Ingredients:

• Grilled chicken breast, sliced

• Fresh spinach leaves

• Sliced strawberries

• Red onion, thinly sliced

• Chopped walnuts or almonds

• Balsamic vinaigrette dressing (choose a low-sodium option)

Instructions:

1. On a plate, arrange fresh spinach leaves, sliced strawberries, red onion, and chopped nuts.

2. Top with grilled chicken slices.

3. Drizzle with balsamic vinaigrette dressing for a sweet and savory salad.

Lentil and Vegetable Stuffed Bell Peppers

Ingredients:

• Bell peppers

• Cooked brown or green lentils

- Mixed vegetables (e.g., zucchini, carrots, celery)

- Onion and garlic, chopped

- Low-sodium vegetable broth

- Tomato sauce

- Fresh herbs (e.g., basil and oregano)

- Salt and pepper to taste

Instructions:

1. Cut the tops off bell peppers and remove the seeds.

2. In a skillet, sauté chopped onion and garlic with mixed vegetables until tender.

3. Add cooked lentils, tomato sauce, and fresh herbs. Season with salt and pepper.

4. Stuff the bell peppers with the lentil and vegetable mixture.

5. Place them in a baking dish with a bit of vegetable broth and bake until the peppers are tender.

Ingredients:

• Cooked quinoa

• Shrimp, peeled and deveined

• Sliced bell peppers

• Chopped broccoli

• Garlic and ginger for flavor

• Low-sodium soy sauce or tamari

• Sesame seeds

Instructions:

1. In a skillet, sauté shrimp with garlic and ginger until they turn pink.

2. Add sliced bell peppers and chopped broccoli. Drizzle with low-sodium soy sauce or tamari and cook until the vegetables are tender.

3. Serve over cooked quinoa and garnish with sesame seeds.

Caprese Wrap

Ingredients:

• Whole-grain wrap or tortilla

• Sliced mozzarella cheese (choose a reduced-fat option)

• Sliced tomatoes

• Fresh basil leaves

• Balsamic glaze

• Olive oil

• Salt and pepper to taste

Instructions:

1. Lay out the whole-grain wrap.

2. Layer with sliced mozzarella cheese, tomatoes, and fresh basil leaves. Drizzle with balsamic glaze and olive oil.

3. Season with salt and pepper. Roll up the wrap for a fresh and simple Caprese flavor.

Ingredients:

• Low-sodium vegetable broth

• Canned low-sodium white beans, drained and rinsed

• Mixed vegetables (e.g., carrots, celery, green beans, spinach)

• Diced tomatoes (canned or fresh)

• Whole wheat pasta or brown rice

• Fresh basil and oregano

• Salt and pepper to taste

Instructions:

1. In a large pot, combine low-sodium vegetable broth, white beans, mixed vegetables, diced tomatoes, and whole wheat pasta or brown rice.

2. Season with fresh basil and oregano, salt, and pepper.

3. Simmer until the vegetables and pasta (or rice) are tender, and enjoy this hearty and heart-healthy soup.

Ingredients:

• 1 cup cooked quinoa

• Cucumber, diced

• Cherry tomatoes, halved

• Kalamata olives, pitted and sliced

• Red onion, finely chopped

• Feta cheese (choose a reduced-fat option)

• Fresh parsley, chopped

• Olive oil and lemon juice for dressing

• Salt and pepper to taste

Instructions:

1. In a bowl, combine cooked quinoa, diced cucumber, cherry tomatoes, Kalamata olives, red onion, crumbled feta cheese, and chopped fresh parsley.

2. Drizzle with a dressing made from olive oil, lemon juice, salt, and pepper.

3. Toss to combine and enjoy this Mediterranean-inspired salad.

Chicken and Avocado Salad with Lime Dressing

Ingredients:

• Grilled chicken breast, sliced

• Mixed salad greens

• Sliced avocado

• Red bell pepper, thinly sliced

• Fresh cilantro leaves

• Lime dressing (lime juice, olive oil, salt, and pepper)

Instructions:

1. On a plate, arrange mixed salad greens, sliced avocado, red bell pepper, and grilled chicken slices.

2. Garnish with fresh cilantro leaves.

3. Drizzle with lime dressing for a refreshing and heart-healthy salad.

Black Bean and Sweet Potato Burrito

Ingredients:

• Whole-grain tortilla

• Baked or roasted sweet potato cubes

• Black beans (canned, drained and rinsed)

• Sliced bell peppers

• Salsa or hot sauce (for added flavor)

• Sliced avocado

Instructions:

1. Fill a whole-grain tortilla with baked or roasted sweet potato cubes, black beans, sliced bell peppers, and salsa or hot sauce.

2. Top with sliced avocado.

3. Roll up the burrito for a hearty and nutritious lunch.

Ingredients:

• Shrimp, peeled and deveined

• Fresh asparagus spears

• Garlic and lemon zest for flavor

• Olive oil

• Salt and pepper to taste

Instructions:

1. In a skillet, sauté shrimp with garlic and lemon zest until they turn pink.

2. Add fresh asparagus spears and continue cooking until they are tender-crisp.

3. Drizzle with a small amount of olive oil and season with salt and pepper.

4. Serve this lemony and garlic-infused dish.

Ingredients:

• Extra-firm tofu, cubed

• Mixed vegetables (e.g., broccoli, snap peas, carrots)

• Low-sodium soy sauce or tamari

• Ginger and garlic for flavor

• Cooked brown rice

Instructions:

1. In a wok or large skillet, stir-fry cubed tofu with ginger and garlic until it's lightly browned.

2. Add mixed vegetables and continue stir-frying until they are tender.

3. Drizzle with low-sodium soy sauce or tamari for flavor.

4. Serve over cooked brown rice for a satisfying and heart-healthy stir-fry.

Baked Salmon with Lemon and Dill

Ingredients:

• Salmon fillets

• Fresh dill

• Lemon slices

• Olive oil

• Salt and pepper to taste

Instructions:

1. Preheat your oven to 375°F (190°C).

2. Place salmon fillets on a baking sheet lined with parchment paper.

3. Drizzle with olive oil, and season with salt and pepper. Top with fresh dill and lemon slices.

4. Bake for about 15-20 minutes, or until the salmon flakes easily with a fork.

Ingredients:

• Spaghetti squash

• Pesto sauce (choose a lower-sodium option)

• Cherry tomatoes, halved

• Fresh basil leaves

• Olive oil

• Parmesan cheese (optional, choose a reduced-fat option)

Instructions:

1. Preheat your oven to 375°F (190°C).

2. Cut the spaghetti squash in half, remove the seeds, and place it cut side down on a baking sheet.

3. Roast the squash for about 30-40 minutes or until the flesh can be easily scraped with a fork to form "noodles."

4. Toss the cooked squash with pesto sauce, cherry tomatoes, fresh basil leaves, a drizzle of olive oil, and Parmesan cheese (if desired).

Grilled Chicken and Quinoa Bowl

Ingredients:

• Grilled chicken breast, sliced

• Cooked quinoa

• Sliced cucumbers

• Sliced red bell peppers

• Hummus (as a spread)

• Greek yogurt and dill sauce (optional)

• Squeeze of lemon juice

• Salt and pepper to taste

Instructions:

1. On a plate, arrange cooked quinoa, grilled chicken slices, sliced cucumbers, and red bell peppers.

2. Spread hummus as a base or drizzle with Greek yogurt and dill sauce.

3. Squeeze fresh lemon juice on top, and season with salt and pepper.

Vegetable and Chickpea Curry

Ingredients:

• Mixed vegetables (e.g., bell peppers, cauliflower, peas)

• Chickpeas (canned, drained and rinsed)

• Onion and garlic, chopped

• Low-sodium vegetable broth

• Curry powder and turmeric

• Cilantro leaves (for garnish)

• Brown rice or whole-grain naan (for serving)

Instructions:

1. In a large pan, sauté chopped onion and garlic until soft.

2. Add mixed vegetables and chickpeas. Season with curry powder and turmeric.

3. Pour in low-sodium vegetable broth and simmer until the vegetables are tender.

4. Serve with brown rice or whole-grain naan and garnish with fresh cilantro leaves.

Grilled Chicken and Veggie Skewers

Ingredients:

• Chicken breast, cubed

• Mixed vegetables (e.g., bell peppers, zucchini, cherry tomatoes)

• Olive oil

• Fresh herbs (e.g., rosemary or thyme)

• Lemon juice

• Salt and pepper to taste

Instructions:

1. Preheat the grill to medium-high heat.

2. Thread chicken and mixed vegetables onto skewers.

3. Brush with olive oil, sprinkle with fresh herbs, and season with salt and pepper.

4. Grill the skewers, turning occasionally, until the chicken is cooked through and the vegetables are tender.

5. Drizzle with lemon juice before serving.

Whole Wheat Pasta with Tomato and Spinach

Ingredients:

• Whole wheat pasta

• Cherry tomatoes, halved

• Fresh spinach leaves

• Garlic, minced

• Olive oil

• Red pepper flakes (optional)

• Fresh basil, chopped

• Salt and pepper to taste

Instructions:

1. Cook whole wheat pasta according to package instructions.

2. In a skillet, sauté minced garlic in olive oil until fragrant.

3. Add cherry tomatoes and cook until they start to soften. Toss in fresh spinach and cook until wilted.

4. Combine with cooked pasta, sprinkle with red pepper flakes (if desired), and season with salt, pepper, and fresh basil.

Grilled Veggie and Quinoa Bowl

Ingredients:

• Cooked quinoa

• Assorted grilled vegetables (e.g., zucchini, bell peppers, asparagus)

• Cherry tomatoes

• Fresh basil leaves

• Balsamic vinegar and olive oil

• Salt and pepper to taste

Instructions:

1. Arrange the grilled vegetables on a plate or in a bowl.

2. Add cooked quinoa and cherry tomatoes. Drizzle with a dressing made from balsamic vinegar and olive oil.

3. Season with salt and pepper and garnish with fresh basil leaves.

Chickpea and Vegetable Stir-Fry

Ingredients:

• Chickpeas (canned, drained and rinsed)

• Mixed vegetables (e.g., broccoli, carrots, snap peas)

• Garlic and ginger for flavor

• Low-sodium soy sauce or tamari

• Cooked brown rice

Instructions:

1. In a wok or large skillet, stir-fry chickpeas, mixed vegetables, garlic, and ginger until the vegetables are tender.

2. Drizzle with low-sodium soy sauce or tamari for flavor.

3. Serve over cooked brown rice for a satisfying and heart-healthy stir-fry.

Baked Lemon Herb Chicken

Ingredients:

• Boneless, skinless chicken breasts

• Fresh lemon juice and zest

• Fresh herbs (e.g., thyme, rosemary, parsley)

• Garlic, minced

• Olive oil

• Salt and pepper to taste

Instructions:

1. Preheat the oven to 375°F (190°C).

2. In a small bowl, combine lemon juice, lemon zest, minced garlic, fresh herbs, and a drizzle of olive oil.

3. Place the chicken breasts in a baking dish. Brush the chicken with the lemon-herb mixture and season with salt and pepper.

4. Bake for about 25-30 minutes or until the chicken is cooked through.

Shrimp and Asparagus Stir-Fry

Ingredients:

• Shrimp, peeled and deveined

• Fresh asparagus spears

• Garlic and ginger for flavor

• Low-sodium soy sauce or tamari

• Red pepper flakes (optional)

• Sesame seeds

Instructions:

1. In a wok or large skillet, stir-fry shrimp with garlic and ginger until they turn pink.

2. Add asparagus spears and continue stir-frying until they are tender-crisp.

3. Drizzle with low-sodium soy sauce or tamari for flavor. Add red pepper flakes if you like some heat.

4. Serve hot, garnished with sesame seeds.

Mediterranean Stuffed Peppers

Ingredients:

• Bell peppers

• Cooked quinoa

• Canned chickpeas, drained and rinsed

• Chopped tomatoes

• Red onion, finely chopped

• Feta cheese (choose a reduced-fat option)

• Fresh parsley, chopped

- Olive oil

- Salt and pepper to taste

Instructions:

1. Preheat the oven to 375°F (190°C).

2. Cut the tops off bell peppers and remove the seeds.

3. In a bowl, combine cooked quinoa, chickpeas, chopped tomatoes, red onion, crumbled feta cheese, and chopped fresh parsley.

4. Stuff the bell peppers with the mixture and place them in a baking dish.

5. Drizzle with a small amount of olive oil, season with salt and pepper, and bake for about 25-30 minutes until the peppers are tender.

Lemon Herb Baked Cod

Ingredients:

- Cod fillets

• Fresh lemon juice and zest

• Fresh herbs (e.g., thyme, rosemary, parsley)

• Garlic, minced

• Olive oil

• Salt and pepper to taste

Instructions:

1. Preheat the oven to 375°F (190°C).

2. In a small bowl, combine lemon juice, lemon zest, minced garlic, fresh herbs, and a drizzle of olive oil.

3. Place the cod fillets on a baking sheet lined with parchment paper. Brush the cod with the lemon-herb mixture and season with salt and pepper.

4. Bake for about 15-20 minutes or until the cod flakes easily with a fork.

Lentil and Vegetable Curry

Ingredients:

• Green or brown lentils

• Mixed vegetables (e.g., carrots, bell peppers, cauliflower)

• Onion, chopped

• Garlic and ginger, minced

• Low-sodium vegetable broth

• Curry powder and turmeric

• Coconut milk (light)

• Fresh cilantro, chopped

• Salt and pepper to taste

Instructions:

1. In a large pot, sauté onions, garlic, and ginger until they soften.

2. Add mixed vegetables, lentils, curry powder, turmeric, and vegetable broth. Simmer until the lentils are tender and the vegetables are cooked.

3. Stir in coconut milk and season with salt and pepper.

4. Garnish with fresh cilantro and serve over brown rice or quinoa.

Spinach and Mushroom Stuffed Chicken Breast

Ingredients:

• Boneless, skinless chicken breasts

• Baby spinach

• Sliced mushrooms

• Garlic, minced

• Olive oil

• Low-sodium chicken broth

• Salt and pepper to taste

Instructions:

1. Preheat the oven to 375°F (190°C).

2. In a skillet, sauté sliced mushrooms and minced garlic in a small amount of olive oil until the mushrooms soften.

3. Add baby spinach and continue to cook until it wilts.

4. Cut a pocket into each chicken breast and stuff with the spinach and mushroom mixture.

5. Season the chicken breasts with salt and pepper.

6. Place them in a baking dish, add a bit of low-sodium chicken broth, and bake for about 25-30 minutes or until the chicken is cooked through.

Quinoa and Black Bean Stuffed Peppers

Ingredients:

• Bell peppers (any color)

• Cooked quinoa

• Canned black beans, drained and rinsed

• Diced tomatoes

• Chopped red onion

• Salsa (choose a low-sodium option)

• Chopped fresh cilantro

• Salt and pepper to taste

Instructions:

1. Preheat the oven to 375°F (190°C).

2. Cut the tops off bell peppers and remove the seeds.

3. In a bowl, combine cooked quinoa, black beans, diced tomatoes, chopped red onion, salsa, and fresh cilantro.

4. Stuff the bell peppers with the mixture, place them in a baking dish, and bake for about 25-30 minutes until the peppers are tender.

Balsamic Glazed Salmon

Ingredients:

• Salmon fillets

• Balsamic vinegar

• Honey or maple syrup

• Dijon mustard

• Minced garlic

• Olive oil

• Salt and pepper to taste

Instructions:

1. In a small bowl, whisk together balsamic vinegar, honey or maple syrup, Dijon mustard, minced garlic, and a drizzle of olive oil.

2. Brush the salmon fillets with the balsamic glaze and season with salt and pepper.

3. Grill or bake the salmon until it flakes easily with a fork, brushing with more glaze as it cooks.

Roasted Vegetable and Chickpea Bowl

Ingredients:

• Assorted roasted vegetables (e.g., sweet potatoes, Brussels sprouts, bell peppers)

• Chickpeas (canned, drained and rinsed)

• Quinoa or brown rice

• Fresh spinach leaves

• Olive oil

• Lemon juice

• Herbs and spices (e.g., rosemary, thyme, paprika)

• Salt and pepper to taste

Instructions:

1. Toss the roasted vegetables and chickpeas with olive oil, herbs, and spices.

2. Serve over cooked quinoa or brown rice, with a bed of fresh spinach.

3. Drizzle with lemon juice and season with salt and pepper.

Tofu and Broccoli Stir-Fry

Ingredients:

• Extra-firm tofu, cubed

• Broccoli florets

• Low-sodium soy sauce or tamari

• Garlic and ginger for flavor

• Cooked brown rice or quinoa

Instructions:

1. In a wok or large skillet, stir-fry cubed tofu with garlic and ginger until lightly browned.

2. Add broccoli florets and continue stir-frying until they're tender. Drizzle with low-sodium soy sauce or tamari.

3. Serve over cooked brown rice or quinoa.

Quinoa and Black Bean Burrito Bowl

Ingredients:

• Cooked quinoa

• Canned black beans, drained and rinsed

• Salsa (choose a low-sodium option)

• Diced avocado

- Fresh cilantro, chopped

- Lime wedges

- Salt and pepper to taste

Instructions:

1. In a bowl, combine cooked quinoa, black beans, salsa, diced avocado, and chopped fresh cilantro.

2. Season with lime juice, salt, and pepper.

3. Create a flavorful burrito bowl to enjoy.

Garlic and Lemon Shrimp with Zoodles

Ingredients:

- Shrimp, peeled and deveined

- Zucchini noodles (zoodles)

- Garlic, minced

- Lemon zest and juice

- Olive oil

• Red pepper flakes (optional)

• Salt and pepper to taste

Instructions:

1. In a skillet, sauté shrimp with garlic and lemon zest until they turn pink.

2. Add zucchini noodles and continue cooking until they're tender. Drizzle with olive oil, lemon juice, and red pepper flakes (if desired).

3. Season with salt and pepper and serve this light and refreshing dish.

Baked Chicken with Spinach and Feta

Ingredients:

• Chicken breasts or thighs

• Fresh spinach leaves

• Reduced-fat feta cheese

• Garlic, minced

• Olive oil

• Salt and pepper to taste

Instructions:

1. Preheat the oven to 375°F (190°C).

2. In a skillet, sauté minced garlic and spinach until the spinach wilts.

3. Cut a pocket into each chicken breast or thigh and stuff with the sautéed spinach and crumbled feta cheese.

4. Place the stuffed chicken in a baking dish, drizzle with olive oil, and season with salt and pepper.

5. Bake for about 25-30 minutes or until the chicken is cooked through.

Mediterranean Chickpea and Quinoa Bowl

Ingredients:

• Cooked quinoa

• Canned chickpeas, drained and rinsed

• Cherry tomatoes, halved

• Cucumber, diced

• Kalamata olives, pitted and sliced

• Red onion, finely chopped

• Feta cheese (choose a reduced-fat option)

• Fresh parsley, chopped

• Olive oil and lemon juice for dressing

• Salt and pepper to taste

Instructions:

1. In a bowl, combine cooked quinoa, chickpeas, cherry tomatoes, cucumber, Kalamata olives, red onion, crumbled feta cheese, and chopped fresh parsley.

2. Drizzle with a dressing made from olive oil, lemon juice, salt, and pepper.

3. Toss to combine and enjoy this Mediterranean-inspired bowl.

Ingredients:

• Chicken breasts or thighs

• Fresh lemon juice and zest

• Garlic, minced

• Olive oil

• Fresh thyme and rosemary, chopped

• Salt and pepper to taste

Instructions:

1. In a bowl, mix lemon juice, lemon zest, minced garlic, chopped fresh herbs, and a drizzle of olive oil.

2. Brush the chicken with the lemon-garlic mixture and season with salt and pepper.

3. Grill until the chicken is cooked through, and it has a delicious citrus and herb flavor.

Black Bean and Vegetable Stir-Fry

Ingredients:

• Canned black beans, drained and rinsed

• Mixed vegetables (e.g., broccoli, bell peppers, snap peas)

• Garlic and ginger for flavor

• Low-sodium soy sauce or tamari

• Cooked brown rice

Instructions:

1. In a wok or large skillet, stir-fry black beans and mixed vegetables with garlic and ginger until the vegetables are tender.

2. Drizzle with low-sodium soy sauce or tamari for flavor.

3. Serve over cooked brown rice for a satisfying and heart-healthy stir-fry.

Quinoa and Spinach Stuffed Portobello Mushrooms

Ingredients:

- Portobello mushrooms

- Cooked quinoa

- Fresh baby spinach

- Garlic, minced

- Olive oil

- Reduced-fat feta cheese

- Salt and pepper to taste

Instructions:

1. Preheat the oven to 375°F (190°C).

2. Remove the stems from the Portobello mushrooms and brush the caps with a small amount of olive oil.

3. In a skillet, sauté minced garlic and baby spinach until the spinach wilts.

4. Mix the sautéed spinach with cooked quinoa and crumbled feta cheese.

5. Stuff the mushroom caps with the quinoa and spinach mixture.

6. Place them on a baking sheet and bake for about 20-25 minutes until the mushrooms are tender.

Seared Tuna with Mango Salsa

Ingredients:

• Ahi tuna steaks

• Mango, diced

• Red bell pepper, diced

• Red onion, finely chopped

• Fresh cilantro, chopped

• Lime juice

• Olive oil

• Salt and pepper to taste

Instructions:

1. Season the tuna steaks with salt and pepper.

2. In a hot skillet, sear the tuna for about 1-2 minutes on each side, depending on your preferred doneness.

3. In a bowl, combine diced mango, red bell pepper, red onion, and fresh cilantro.

4. Drizzle with lime juice and a touch of olive oil.

5. Serve the seared tuna topped with the refreshing mango salsa.

Mixed Berry Parfait

Ingredients:

• Greek yogurt (choose a low-fat or non-fat option)

• Mixed berries (e.g., strawberries, blueberries, raspberries)

• Honey or agave nectar

• Granola (choose a low-sugar, whole-grain option)

Instructions:

1. In a glass or bowl, layer Greek yogurt, mixed berries, and a drizzle of honey or agave nectar.

2. Top with a sprinkle of granola for added crunch and sweetness.

Chocolate-Dipped Strawberries

Ingredients:

• Fresh strawberries

• Dark chocolate (70% cocoa or higher)

• Chopped nuts (e.g., almonds, walnuts)

Instructions:

1. Melt dark chocolate in a microwave-safe bowl in short intervals or using a double boiler.

2. Dip fresh strawberries in the melted chocolate.

3. Sprinkle with chopped nuts while the chocolate is still soft.

4. Place on a tray lined with parchment paper and let them cool until the chocolate hardens.

Baked Apples with Cinnamon and Walnuts

Ingredients:

• Apples (choose a heart-healthy variety like Granny Smith)

• Cinnamon

• Chopped walnuts

• Honey (optional)

Instructions:

1. Preheat the oven to 375°F (190°C).

2. Core the apples, leaving the bottoms intact. Sprinkle with cinnamon and fill the center with chopped walnuts.

3. Optionally, drizzle with a touch of honey.

4. Bake for about 20-25 minutes or until the apples are tender.

Chia Seed Pudding with Berries

Ingredients:

• Chia seeds

• Unsweetened almond milk (or any milk of your choice)

• Fresh berries (e.g., blueberries, raspberries)

• Honey (optional)

• Vanilla extract

Instructions:

1. In a bowl, mix chia seeds, almond milk, a drop of vanilla extract, and a drizzle of honey if desired.

2. Stir well and refrigerate for a few hours or overnight until it thickens.

3. Top with fresh berries before serving.

Grilled Pineapple with Yogurt and Honey

Ingredients:

• Pineapple slices

• Greek yogurt (choose a low-fat or non-fat option)

• Honey

• Fresh mint leaves (optional)

Instructions:

1. Grill pineapple slices until they have grill marks and are slightly caramelized.

2. Serve with a dollop of Greek yogurt.

3. Drizzle with honey and garnish with fresh mint leaves for a delightful and heart-healthy dessert.

Ingredients:

• Low-fat Greek yogurt

• Mixed berries (e.g., strawberries, blueberries, blackberries)

• Honey or agave nectar

• Almond slices (or any preferred nuts)

Instructions:

1. In a glass or bowl, layer low-fat Greek yogurt, mixed berries, and a drizzle of honey or agave nectar.

2. Top with almond slices or your favorite nuts for added texture and flavor.

Frozen Banana Pops

Ingredients:

• Ripe bananas, peeled and cut in half

• Low-sugar dark chocolate (70% cocoa or higher)

• Chopped nuts (e.g., almonds, pistachios)

• Popsicle sticks

Instructions:

1. Insert popsicle sticks into the cut end of each banana half. Melt dark chocolate and dip the bananas.

2. Quickly sprinkle with chopped nuts while the chocolate is still soft.

3. Place on a tray lined with parchment paper and freeze until firm.

Watermelon Granita

Ingredients:

• Watermelon, cubed and seedless

• Lime juice

• Fresh mint leaves (optional)

Instructions:

1. Blend cubed watermelon and lime juice until smooth. Pour into a shallow dish and freeze.

2. Every 30 minutes, scrape with a fork until you achieve a granita-like texture.

3. Serve in small bowls, garnished with fresh mint leaves if desired.

Mixed Fruit Salad with Citrus Glaze

Ingredients:

• A variety of fresh fruits (e.g., orange segments, grapefruit, kiwi, strawberries)

• Fresh mint leaves

• Lime juice

• Honey or agave nectar

Instructions:

1. In a bowl, combine your choice of fresh fruits.

2. Drizzle with a citrus glaze made from lime juice and honey or agave nectar.

3. Garnish with fresh mint leaves for a refreshing and heart-healthy dessert.

Baked Pears with Cinnamon and Walnuts

Ingredients:

• Ripe pears, halved and cored

• Cinnamon

• Chopped walnuts

• Honey or maple syrup

Instructions:

1. Preheat the oven to 375°F (190°C).

2. Place pear halves, cut side up, in a baking dish.

3. Sprinkle with cinnamon, chopped walnuts, and drizzle with honey or maple syrup.

4. Bake for about 20-25 minutes or until the pears are tender and caramelized.

Dark Chocolate-Dipped Banana Bites

Ingredients:

• Ripe bananas, sliced into bite-sized pieces

• Dark chocolate (70% cocoa or higher)

• Chopped nuts (e.g., almonds, walnuts)

• Unsweetened shredded coconut

Instructions:

1. Melt dark chocolate in a microwave-safe bowl or using a double boiler.

2. Dip banana pieces in the melted chocolate.

3. Sprinkle with chopped nuts and shredded coconut while the chocolate is still soft.

4. Place on a tray lined with parchment paper and let them cool until the chocolate hardens.

Frozen Yogurt Bark

Ingredients:

- Greek yogurt (choose low-fat or non-fat)

- Fresh berries (e.g., strawberries, blueberries)

- Honey or agave nectar

- Unsweetened shredded coconut

Instructions:

1. Spread Greek yogurt onto a parchment paper-lined baking sheet.

2. Add fresh berries, drizzle with honey or agave nectar, and sprinkle with shredded coconut.

3. Freeze until firm, then break into pieces and enjoy.

Mango Sorbet

Ingredients:

1. Ripe mangoes, peeled, pitted, and diced

2. Lime juice

3. Honey or agave nectar

Instructions:

1. Blend ripe mangoes, lime juice, and honey or agave nectar until smooth.

2. Pour the mixture into a container and freeze until it reaches a sorbet-like consistency.

3. Serve chilled for a refreshing, heart-healthy dessert.

Chia Seed Pudding with Berries and Almonds

Ingredients:

• Chia seeds

• Unsweetened almond milk (or any milk of your choice)

• Fresh berries (e.g., blueberries, raspberries)

• Sliced almonds

• Honey (optional)

• Vanilla extract

Instructions:

1. In a bowl, mix chia seeds, almond milk, a drop of vanilla extract, and a drizzle of honey if desired.

2. Stir well and refrigerate for a few hours or overnight until it thickens.

3. Top with fresh berries and sliced almonds before serving.

Peach and Berry Crisp

Ingredients:

• Ripe peaches, sliced

• Mixed berries (e.g., blueberries, raspberries)

• Oats

• Almond flour

• Chopped almonds

• Cinnamon

• Honey or maple syrup

Instructions:

1. Preheat the oven to 375°F (190°C).

2. In a bowl, mix sliced peaches and mixed berries.

3. In a separate bowl, combine oats, almond flour, chopped almonds, and cinnamon.

4. Spread the fruit mixture in a baking dish and top with the oat mixture. Drizzle with honey or maple syrup.

5. Bake for about 30-35 minutes or until the topping is golden and the fruit is bubbling.

Apple and Cinnamon Baked Oatmeal

Ingredients:

• Rolled oats

• Apples, peeled, cored, and diced

• Cinnamon

• Unsweetened applesauce

• Unsweetened almond milk (or any milk of your choice)

• Honey or maple syrup (optional)

Instructions:

1. Preheat the oven to 375°F (190°C).

2. In a baking dish, combine rolled oats, diced apples, and a dash of cinnamon. Mix in unsweetened applesauce and unsweetened almond milk.

3. Optionally, drizzle with honey or maple syrup for added sweetness.

4. Bake for about 30-35 minutes or until the oatmeal is cooked through and the top is golden.

Mixed Berry and Almond Chia Pudding

Ingredients:

• Chia seeds

• Unsweetened almond milk (or any milk of your choice)

• Mixed berries (e.g., strawberries, blueberries, raspberries)

• Sliced almonds

• Honey or agave nectar

• Vanilla extract

Instructions:

1. In a bowl, mix chia seeds, almond milk, a drop of vanilla extract, and a drizzle of honey or agave nectar if desired.

2. Stir well and refrigerate for a few hours or overnight until it thickens.

3. Layer with mixed berries and top with sliced almonds before serving.

Banana and Walnut Ice Cream

Ingredients:

• Ripe bananas, sliced and frozen

• Chopped walnuts

• Cinnamon

• Honey (optional)

Instructions:

1. Blend frozen banana slices until smooth and creamy. Mix in chopped walnuts and a dash of cinnamon.

2. Optionally, drizzle with honey for added sweetness.

3. Serve immediately or freeze briefly for a firmer texture.

Chocolate Avocado Mousse

Ingredients:

• Ripe avocados

• Unsweetened cocoa powder

• Honey or agave nectar

• Vanilla extract

• Unsweetened almond milk (or any milk of your choice)

Instructions:

1. In a blender, combine ripe avocados, unsweetened cocoa powder, honey or agave nectar, a drop of vanilla extract, and a splash of almond milk.

2. Blend until smooth and creamy.

3. Chill in the refrigerator and serve as a rich and healthy chocolate mousse.

Ingredients:

• Kiwis, peeled and sliced

• Strawberries, hulled and halved

• Lemon juice

• Honey or agave nectar

Instructions:

1. Blend kiwis, strawberries, lemon juice, and honey or agave nectar until smooth.

2. Pour the mixture into a container and freeze until it reaches a sorbet-like consistency.

3. Enjoy a refreshing and heart-healthy sorbet.

CHAPTER THREE

CONCLUSION

In conclusion, maintaining a heart-healthy diet and lifestyle is a journey filled with choices that can significantly impact our cardiovascular well-being. By adopting the principles of moderation and balance, understanding how to read and interpret nutrition labels, and making informed choices when it comes to fats in recipes, we empower ourselves to take control of our heart health.

A heart-healthy diet is not about deprivation but about mindful and informed choices. It encompasses the careful selection of nutrient-rich foods, the avoidance of excessive saturated and trans fats, and the reduction of added sugars. It also extends beyond the plate, encompassing regular exercise, effective stress management, and the importance of adequate sleep.

By embracing these principles and practices, we can reduce the risk of heart disease, support overall health, and savor the joys of a balanced and nutritious diet. Each step taken towards moderation, education, and mindful eating brings us closer to a healthier heart, improved well-being, and a better quality of life. Ultimately, by making heart-healthy choices a part of our everyday routine, we contribute to a healthier, happier, and more vibrant future for ourselves and our loved ones.